Spina Bifida: Health and Development Across the Life Course

Guest Editors

MARK E. SWANSON, MD, MPH
ADRIAN D. SANDLER, MD

PEDIATRIC CLINICS
OF NORTH AMERICA

www.pediatric.theclinics.com

August 2010 • Volume 57 • Number 4

SAUNDERS an imprint of ELSEVIER, Inc.

W.B. SAUNDERS COMPANY
A Division of Elsevier Inc.

1600 John F. Kennedy Boulevard • Suite 1800 • Philadelphia, Pennsylvania 19103-2899

http://www.theclinics.com

THE PEDIATRIC CLINICS OF NORTH AMERICA Volume 57, Number 4
August 2010 ISSN 0031-3955, ISBN-13: 978-1-4377-2477-6

Editor: Carla Holloway
Developmental Editor: Theresa Collier

The Pediatric Clinics of North America (ISSN 0031-3955) is published bimonthly by Elsevier Inc., 360 Park Avenue South, New York, NY 10010-1710. Months of issue are February, April, June, August, October, and December. Periodicals postage paid at New York, NY and additional mailing offices. Subscription prices are $167.00 per year (US individuals), $378.00 per year (US institutions), $227.00 per year (Canadian individuals), $503.00 per year (Canadian institutions), $270.00 per year (international individuals), $503.00 per year (international institutions), $83.00 per year (US students and residents), and $142.00 per year (international and Canadian residents and students). To receive students/resident rare, orders must be accompanied by name of affiliated institution, date of term, and the signature of program/residency coordinator on institution letterhead. Orders will be billed at individual rate until proof of status is received. Foreign air speed delivery is included in all *Clinics* subscription prices. All prices are subject to change without notice. **POSTMASTER:** Send address changes to *The Pediatric Clinics of North America*, Elsevier Health Sciences Division, Subscription Customer Service, 3251 Riverport Lane, Maryland Heights, MO 63043. **Customer Service: 1-800-654-2452 (US and Canada). From outside of the US and Canada: 1-314-447-8871. Fax: 1-314-447-8029. For print support, E-mail: JournalsCustomerService-usa@elsevier.com. For online support, E-mail: JournalsOnlineSupport-usa@elsevier.com.**

Reprints. For copies of 100 or more, of articles in this publication, please contact the Commercial Reprints Department, Elsevier Inc., 360 Park Avenue South, New York, NY 10010-1710. Tel.: 212-633-3812; Fax: 212-462-1935; E-mail: reprints@elsevier.com.

The Pediatric Clinics of North America is also published in Spanish by McGraw-Hill Inter-americana Editores S.A., Mexico City, Mexico; in Portuguese by Riechmann and Affonso Editores, Rua Comandante Coelho 1085, CEP 21250, Rio de Janeiro, Brazil; and in Greek by Althayia SA, Athens, Greece.

The Pediatric Clinics of North America is covered in *MEDLINE/PubMed (Index Medicus), Excerpta Medica, Current Contents, Current Contents/Clinical Medicine, Science Citation Index, ASCA, ISI/BIOMED,* and *BIOSIS.*

Printed in the United States of America.

418-92
ped
2019
v. 57
no. 4

GOAL STATEMENT

The goal of *Pediatric Clinics of North America* is to keep practicing physicians up to date with current clinical practice in pediatrics by providing timely articles reviewing the state of the art in patient care.

ACCREDITATION

The *Pediatric Clinics of North America* is planned and implemented in accordance with the Essential Areas and Policies of the Accreditation Council for Continuing Medical Education (ACCME) through the joint sponsorship of the University Of Virginia School Of Medicine and Elsevier. The University Of Virginia School of Medicine is accredited by the ACCME to provide continuing medical education for physicians.

The University of Virginia School of Medicine designates this educational activity for a maximum of 15 *AMA PRA Category 1 Credits*™ for each issue, 90 credits per year. Physicians should only claim credit commensurate with the extent of their participation in the activity.

The American Medical Association has determined that physicians not licensed in the US who participate in this CME activity are eligible for a maximum of 15 *AMA PRA Category 1 Credits*™ for each issue, 90 credits per year.

Credit can be earned by reading the text material, taking the CME examination online at http://www.theclinics.com/home/cme, and completing the evaluation. After taking the test, you will be required to review any and all incorrect answers. Following completion of the test and evaluation, your credit will be awarded and you may print your certificate.

FACULTY DISCLOSURE/CONFLICT OF INTEREST

The University of Virginia School of Medicine, as an ACCME accredited provider, endorses and strives to comply with the Accreditation Council for Continuing Medical Education (ACCME) Standards of Commercial Support, Commonwealth of Virginia statutes, University of Virginia policies and procedures, and associated federal and private regulations and guidelines on the need for disclosure and monitoring of proprietary and financial interests that may affect the scientific integrity and balance of content delivered in continuing medical education activities under our auspices.

The University of Virginia School of Medicine requires that all CME activities accredited through this institution be developed independently and be scientifically rigorous, balanced and objective in the presentation/discussion of its content, theories and practices.

All authors/editors participating in an accredited CME activity are expected to disclose to the readers relevant financial relationships with commercial entities occurring within the past 12 months (such as grants or research support, employee, consultant, stock holder, member of speakers bureau, etc.). The University of Virginia School of Medicine will employ appropriate mechanisms to resolve potential conflicts of interest to maintain the standards of fair and balanced education to the reader. Questions about specific strategies can be directed to the Office of Continuing Medical Education, University of Virginia School of Medicine, Charlottesville, Virginia.

The faculty and staff of the University of Virginia Office of Continuing Medical Education have no financial affiliations to disclose.

The authors/editors listed below have identified no financial or professional relationships for themselves or their spouse/partner:

Elizabeth Adams, PhD, RD; Ann I. Alriksson-Schmidt, PhD, MSPH; Melissa H. Bellin, PhD, MSW, LCSW; Cecily L. Betz, PhD, RN, FAAN; Patricia G. Braun, DNSc, MSN, MA, CPNP, RNC; Carley Butler, ACSW; Jill Caruso; Amy Colgan-Niemeyer, CPT, CES; Katie A. Devine, PhD; Brad E. Dicianno, MD; Kurt A. Freeman, PhD; Carla Holloway, (Acquisitions Editor); Grayson N. Holmbeck, PhD; Susan R. Leibold, RN, MSN, CNS-P, CDDN; Kristy Macias; Stacey Mizokawa, PhD; Ann Neville-Jan, PhD, OTR/L, FAOTA; Karen Rheuban, MD (Test Author); Adrian D. Sandler, MD (Guest Editor); Kathleen J. Sawin, PhD, CPNP-PC; Jamie Smith; Kathryn Smith, RN, MN; Mark E. Swanson, MD, MPH (Guest Editor); Judy K. Thibadeau, RN, MN; and T. Andrew Zabel, PhD, ABPP.

The authors/editors listed below identified the following professional or financial affiliations for themselves or their spouse/partner:

Andrea D. Fairman, MOT, OTR/L, CPRP is employed by The University of Pittsburgh and AOT, Inc; and is a consultant for The University of Pittsburgh and the Centers for Disease Control.

Shannon B. Juengst, MS, CRC is employed by The University of Pittsburgh and is a consultant for the Centers for Disease Control.

Ronna Linroth, PhD, OT is employed by Gillette Children's Specialty Healthcare.

Bambang Parmanto, PhD is employed by The University of Pittsburgh.

Disclosure of Discussion of Non-FDA Approved Uses for Pharmaceutical Products and/or Medical Devices

The University of Virginia School of Medicine, as an ACCME provider, requires that all faculty presenters identify and disclose any off-label uses for pharmaceutical and medical device products. The University of Virginia School of Medicine recommends that each physician fully review all the available data on new products or procedures prior to clinical use.

TO ENROLL

To enroll in the Pediatric Clinics of North America Continuing Medical Education program, call customer service at 1-800-654-2452 or visit us online at www.theclinics.com/home/cme. The CME program is available to subscribers for an additional fee of $223.00.

Contributors

GUEST EDITORS

MARK E. SWANSON, MD, MPH
Senior Medical Adviser, Division of Human Development and Disability, National Center on Birth Defects and Developmental Disabilities, Centers for Disease Control and Prevention, Atlanta, Georgia

ADRIAN D. SANDLER, MD
Medical Director, Olson Huff Center, Mission Children's Hospital, Asheville, North Carolina; Adjunct Associate Professor, Department of Pediatrics, University of North Carolina at Chapel Hill, Chapel Hill, North Carolina

AUTHORS

ANN I. ALRIKSSON-SCHMIDT, PhD, MSPH
Senior Service Fellow/Health Scientist, Division of Human Development and Disability, National Center on Birth Defects and Developmental Disabilities, Centers for Disease Control and Prevention, Atlanta, Georgia

ELIZABETH ADAMS, PhD, RD
Assistant Professor, Department of Public Health and Preventive Medicine, Oregon Health and Science University, Portland, Oregon

MELISSA H. BELLIN, PhD, MSW, LCSW
Assistant Professor and Chair of Health Specialization, University of Maryland, School of Social Work, Baltimore, Maryland

CECILY L. BETZ, PhD, RN, FAAN
Associate Professor of Clinical Pediatrics, Keck School of Medicine, Department of Pediatrics; Director of Nursing Training and Director of Research, USC Center for Excellence in Developmental Disabilities, Childrens Hospital Los Angeles, University of Southern California, Los Angeles, California

PATRICIA G. BRAUN, DNSc, MSN, MA, CPNP, RNC
Assistant Professor, Northern Illinois University, DeKalb, Illinois

CARLEY BUTLER, ACSW
USC Center of Excellence in Developmental Disabilities, Children's Hospital Los Angeles, Los Angeles, California

JILL CARUSO
Spina Bifida Association of America, Monroe, Michigan

AMY COLGAN-NIEMEYER, CPT, CES
Spina Bifida Association of America, Saint George, Utah

KATIE A. DEVINE, PhD
Post-Doctoral Fellow, Department of Psychology, Loyola University Chicago, Chicago, Illinois

BRAD E. DICIANNO, MD
Assistant Professor, Department of Veterans Affairs, Human Engineering Research Laboratories (HERL), Veterans Affairs Pittsburgh Healthcare System; Department of Physical Medicine and Rehabilitation, University of Pittsburgh Medical Center (UPMC), Pittsburgh, Pennsylvania

ANDREA D. FAIRMAN, MOT, OTR/L, CPRP
Occupational Therapist, PhD Candidate, Department of Rehabilitation Science and Technology, University of Pittsburgh, School of Health and Rehabilitation Sciences, Pittsburgh, Pennsylvania; Department of Physical Medicine and Rehabilitation, Adult Spina Bifida Clinic, University of Pittsburgh Medical Center (UPMC), Pittsburgh, Pennsylvania

KURT A. FREEMAN, PhD
Associate Professor of Pediatrics and Psychiatry, Director of Training, Division of Psychology, Child Development and Rehabilitation Center, Oregon Health and Science University, Portland, Oregon

GRAYSON N. HOLMBECK, PhD
Professor and Director of Clinical Training, Department of Psychology, Loyola University Chicago, Chicago, Illinois

SHANNON B. JUENGST, MS, CRC
Pre-Doctoral Student/Research Specialist, Department of Occupational Therapy, University of Pittsburgh, School of Health and Rehabilitation Sciences, Pittsburgh, Pennsylvania

SUSAN R. LEIBOLD, RN, MSN, CNS-P, CDDN
Developmental Disabilities, Texas Scottish Rite Hospital for Children, Dallas, Texas

RONNA LINROTH, PhD, OT
Operations Manger, Gillette Lifetime Specialty Healthcare Clinic, Gillette Children's Specialty Healthcare, St. Paul, Minnesota

KRISTY MACIAS
University Center for Excellence in Developmental Disabilities, Children's Hospital Los Angeles, University of Southern California, Los Angeles, California

STACEY MIZOKAWA, PhD
Psychologist, University Center for Excellence in Developmental Disabilities, Childrens Hospital Los Angeles, University of Southern California, Los Angeles, California

ANN NEVILLE-JAN, PhD, OTR/L, FAOTA
Associate Chair (Faculty and Curriculum), Associate Professor, Department of Occupational Science and Occupational Therapy, University of Southern California, Los Angeles, California

BAMBANG PARMANTO, PhD
Associate Professor, Department of Health Information Management, University of Pittsburgh School of Health and Rehabilitation Sciences, Pittsburgh, Pennsylvania

ADRIAN D. SANDLER, MD
Medical Director, Olson Huff Center, Mission Children's Hospital, Asheville, North Carolina; Adjunct Associate Professor, Department of Pediatrics, University of North Carolina at Chapel Hill, Chapel Hill, North Carolina

JAMIE SMITH
Spina Bifida Support Group of Arkansas, Bentonville, Arkansas

KATHRYN SMITH, RN, MN
Associate Director for Administration, University Center for Excellence in Developmental Disabilities, University of Southern California, Los Angeles, California; Co-Director, Spina Bifida Center, Childrens Hospital Los Angeles, Los Angeles, California; Professor of Pediatrics, Keck School of Medicine University Southern California, Los Angeles, California

MARK E. SWANSON, MD, MPH
Senior Medical Adviser, Division of Human Development and Disability, National Center on Birth Defects and Developmental Disabilities, Centers for Disease Control and Prevention, Atlanta, Georgia

KATHLEEN J. SAWIN, PhD, CPNP-PC, FAAN
Professor and Research Chair in the Nursing of Children, A Position jointly sponsored by the College of Nursing, Children's Hospital of Wisconsin, Center Scientist, Self-Management Science Center College of Nursing, University of Wisconsin-Milwaukee, Milwaukee, Wisconsin

JUDY K. THIBADEAU, RN, MN
Health Scientist, Division of Human Development and Disability, National Center on Birth Defects and Developmental Disabilities, Centers for Disease Control and Prevention, Atlanta, Georgia

T. ANDREW ZABEL, PhD, ABPP
Neuropsychologist, Department of Neuropsychology, Philip A. Keelty Center for Spina Bifida and Related Conditions, Kennedy Krieger Institute; Assistant Professor, Department of Psychiatry and Behavioral Science, Johns Hopkins University School of Medicine, Baltimore, Maryland

Contents

> Spina bifida is the most common of the neural tube defects, which include myelomeningocele, encephalocele, and anencephaly. Spina bifida is a complex and multisystem birth defect, in which one or more vertebral arches may be incomplete. This article discusses the sensory and motor impairments, neurologic disorders, orthopedic and cognitive impairments, and skin and other problems associated with spina bifida. This article also summarizes some of the key clinical issues in the care of children with this complex birth defect.

> Because children with chronic conditions, such as spina bifida, have grown up into adults in increasing numbers, they and their families have increasingly questioned whether they have reached their full potential and maximized their participation in adult activities. Lack of knowledgeable adult medical providers and longitudinal data about natural history places more responsibility on individuals and their family for self-care of the impairment. This article describes the need for the life course model, which merges several concepts and principles related to children with disabilities and provides a framework for services and research to achieve the desired adult outcomes.

> This article outlines and summarizes the rationale and the working process that was undertaken by the National Spina Bifida Program to address the issues of transitioning throughout the life course for persons growing up with spina bifida. Their challenges include achieving independent living, vocational independence, community mobility, and participation in social activities, and health management. The creation, the underlying concepts, and the dissemination of the Life Course Model are described.

> The transition of youth with spina bifida into adulthood is an exciting opportunity to branch out, explore and participate in community, and

The Life Course Model facilitates a developmental approach to assessment and intervention along life's trajectory. This Life Course Model provides information about key developmental milestones for particular age groups, validated assessments that can be performed by clinicians or teachers to determine if milestones have been reached, useful suggestions for intervening in creative ways at each step, and evidence-based references. In this article, the authors introduce the viewpoints of several key clinicians who are involved in the care of individuals with spina bifida and how the Life Course Model can assist them, their patients, and their families in the process of assessment, intervention, collaboration with other clinicians, and follow-up. A case study is used to demonstrate the experience of comprehensive and collaborative management in transitioning a child and his family from infancy to adulthood.

This article describes the utility of a spina bifida-specific electronic medical record (SB EMR). Standardization and pooling of data through the SB EMR will facilitate development of increased knowledge for advancing interventions for SB treatment, rehabilitation, and support. Integration with a Web-based transition tool will enhance the efficiency and efficacy of interventions delivered by clinicians. The SB EMR may also be used by SB clinic staff to manage and monitor the developmental course SB through childhood and the adolescent years. Further, implementation of the SB EMR in conjunction with the life-course model will assist in the transition of young persons with SB to adult roles.

Based on the experience of 2 physicians from physiatry and developmental pediatrics, this article proposes a framework for improving care and outcomes for children with spina bifida. The combined skills of physiatrists and developmental pediatricians, along with other disciplines, can form the ideal team to manage the complex issues faced by this population. The developmental pediatrician is best suited for directing care for younger children through the elementary and middle school years, during which time behavioral and educational issues are prominent. As the child assumes more responsibility for self-management in adolescence, the physiatrist is ideally suited to provide major clinical input that improves functional outcomes. The addition of the discipline of physiatry to traditional, developmentally oriented pediatric interdisciplinary teams can add the much needed dimensions of activity and participation, and improve functional outcomes at the adult level by encouraging activities in adolescence that lead to full participation in adulthood.

others. The United States is increasingly multicultural and diverse, and it is becoming more difficult to categorize individuals into a single racial/ethnic group. This article uses the term ethnicity as defined by the Institute of Medicine and avoids using race unless part of a particular study.

In this article an agenda is discussed for further research, services, and program development identified in the development of the Life Course Model Web site for individuals with spina bifida, their families and the health care providers who work with them. The gaps identified during development of the Life Course Model Web site revealed that there has been minimal progress made on the research agenda since the 2003 consensus document, "Evidence-Based Practice in Spina Bifida: Developing a Research Agenda" or the summary document from the First World Congress on Spina Bifida Research and Care gathering, "The Future is Now," in 2009. Gaps are delineated in the three main areas of the transition curriculum (self-management/health, personal and social relationships, and employment/income support), and recommendations for future research and program development are proposed.

FORTHCOMING ISSUES

October 2010
Birthmarks of Medical Significance
Beth A. Drolet, MD, and
Maria C. Garzon, MD,
Guest Editors

December 2010
Pediatric Chest Pain
Guy D. Eslick, PhD, and
Steven Selbst, MD, *Guest Editors*

February 2011
Pediatric and Adolescent
Psychopharmacology
Donald E. Greydanus, MD, FAAP, FSAM,
FIAP (HON), Dilip R. Patel MD, FAAP,
FSAM, FAACPDM, FACSM, and
Cynthia Feucht, Pharm D, BCPS,
Guest Editors

April 2011
Sleep in Children and Adolescents
Judith Owens, MD, MPH
and Jodi A. Mindell, PhD,
Guest Editors

RECENT ISSUES

June 2010
Adolescents and Sports
Dilip R. Patel, MD, FAAP, FACSM,
FAACPDM, FSAM, and
Donald E. Greydanus, MD, FAAP,
FSAM, FIAP (H),
Guest Editors

April 2010
Optimization of Outcomes for Children
After Solid Organ Transplantation
Vicky Lee Ng, MD, FRCPC, and
Sandy Feng, MD, PhD, *Guest Editors*

February 2010
Hematopoietic Stem Cell Transplantation
Max J. Coppes, MD, PhD, MBA,
Terry J. Fry, MD, and
Crystal L. Mackall, MD,
Guest Editors

RELATED INTEREST

Pediatric Clinics of North America Volume 55, Issues 5 and 6 (October and December 2008)
Developmental Disabilities, Parts I and II
Donald E. Greydanus, MD, FAAP, FSAM, FIAP (HON), Dilip R. Patel, MD, FAAP, FSAM, FAACPDM, FACSM, and Helen Pratt, PhD, *Guest Editors*
www.pediatric.theclinics.com

THE CLINICS ARE NOW AVAILABLE ONLINE!

Access your subscription at:
www.theclinics.com

Preface

Spina Bifida

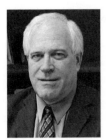   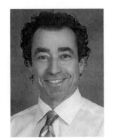

Mark E. Swanson, MD, MPH   Adrian D. Sandler, MD
Guest Editors

Spina bifida is one of the most recognized impairments in pediatrics. Children with open lesions of the spine are identified increasingly in utero and always at birth, setting the stage for a lifelong journey to adulthood for the child and the family. Planning for services and supports requires input from an interdisciplinary team of professionals, working closely with the child, parents, and family members. With life expectancy stretching well into the fourth decade and beyond, the approach to childhood service delivery needs to be one that considers the entire life course. Principles of child development and the International Classification of Functioning, Disability and Health offer two complementary approaches to guide services and supports.

In this issue of *Pediatric Clinic of North America*, we discuss the natural history of spina bifida and the challenges and opportunities for improving health and development during childhood. There is a focus on the desired outcome of optimal function, independence, and full community participation for adults with spina bifida. The key role to be played by pediatricians and other health professionals is emphasized.

The Spina Bifida Transition Working Group was formed under the direction of the Centers for Disease Control and Prevention in 2006. Most of the authors of this issue were part of the Working Group that produced the Life Course Model for Spina Bifida, a web-based resource of goals (and the methods to reach them) across the life course in three important domains of life. The Working Group identified pertinent and pressing health and developmental issues at each stage of childhood in three domains: health/self-management, relationships, and education/income support. Successful navigation across the life course in these domains by individuals with spina bifida offers the best opportunity for successful adult life. The Life Course Model provides a framework for clinical service delivery and future research and is a resource for families and clinicians alike.

Sandler's overview article on current topics in spina bifida sets the stage for this journal issue. The conceptual framework for the Life Course Model is discussed in the article by Swanson. This formed the base for the development of the model.

Pediatr Clin N Am 57 (2010) xv–xvi
doi:10.1016/j.pcl.2010.08.005
0031-3955/10/$ — see front matter © 2010 Elsevier Inc. All rights reserved.
pediatric.theclinics.com

Thibadeau and Alriksson-Schmidt discuss how the Working Group formed and took on the task of creating a Web site. The design of the Web site and examples of the content are in the Zabel article.

A series of articles by Holmbeck, Betz, and Dicianno discuss the usefulness of the Life Course Model Web site from the perspective of the family, individual, and clinician. Participation by all three stakeholder groups in using the model offers great promise for synergy in the implementation of the model.

The Fairman article addresses how the components of the model can be integrated into an electronic medical record (EMR). The EMR can be a repository of the developmental and health information that tracks a child's trajectory.

Developmental pediatrics' strengths in spina bifida care are compared to and contrasted with the strengths of physiatry in the article by Swanson and Dicianno. The article concludes with a discussion on how these approaches can complement each other and lead to better health outcomes.

This issue also addresses two important issues that are included in the Life Course Model but merit special emphasis: 1) bowel and bladder continence (Leibold; Smith and colleagues), because of the far-reaching effects of continence on health and quality of life; and 2) cultural issues (Smith and colleagues), which should be addressed in every clinical setting but have increased importance with changing demographics of the spina bifida population.

Last, Sawin's article discusses the most pressing needs for acquiring new knowledge to establish the evidence base on how to deliver improved health, developmental, and educational services to achieve desired outcomes, as described in the Life Course Model. Much of the content in the model was based on expert consensus and extrapolation from other impairments. Significant work remains to fill in the gaps and provide solid guidance for care that will establish a successful trajectory to successful adult life for those living with spina bifida. The Life Course Model will be available on www.spinabifidaassociation.org in late 2010 or directly at www.spinabifidatransitioning.org.

Mark E. Swanson, MD, MPH
Division of Human Development and Disability
National Center on Birth Defects and Developmental Disabilities
Centers for Disease Control and Prevention
1600 Clifton Road, Atlanta, GA 30333, USA

Adrian D. Sandler, MD
Department of Pediatrics
University of North Carolina School of Medicine
Chapel Hill, NC 27599, USA

Olson Huff Center, Mission Children's Hospital
11 Vanderbilt Park Drive
Asheville, NC 28803, USA

E-mail addresses:
cfu9@cdc.gov (M.E. Swanson)
adsandler@pol.net (A.D. Sandler)

Children with Spina Bifida: Key Clinical Issues

Adrian D. Sandler, MD[a,b,]*

KEYWORDS

• Spina bifida • Myelomeningocele • Hydrocephalus • Treatment

Spina bifida is the most common of the neural tube defects (NTDs), which include myelomeningocele, encephalocele, and anencephaly. Spina bifida occulta is a common spectrum condition, present in approximately 5% of the population, in which one or more vertebral arches may be incomplete (**Fig. 1**). The spinal cord is normal, and there are usually no associated neurologic abnormalities. Spina bifida occulta may be accompanied by localized skin abnormalities (dermal sinus, dimples, and pigmented or hairy skin). If there is an associated skin-covered swelling, with an intact spinal cord, the terms meningocele or lipomeningocele are used. Meningoceles are almost always present in the lumbosacral area. A lipomeningocele may be entirely asymptomatic, but intraspinal lipomas can impinge on the cord and lead to progressive weakness and/or deformity.

When spina bifida is open and associated with a malformed spinal cord and a sac, the terms myelomeningocele or meningomyelocele are used. Myelomeningoceles arise as a consequence of incomplete or disrupted neurulation during the fourth week of gestation, when the embryo is only 3 to 5 mm in length (**Fig. 2**).[1] The myelomeningocele includes the splayed-open malformed cord (neural placode) as well as the meninges and fatty tissue (**Fig. 3**). Myelomeningoceles are often intact, with a meningeal sac enclosing cerebrospinal fluid (CSF), but in many cases the sac is disrupted and leaking CSF at birth. Myelomeningoceles vary in size and location, and the range of associated motor and sensory impairments depends on the level of the lesion.

SENSORY AND MOTOR IMPAIRMENTS

Spinal level is determined by careful examination of sensation and motor function, and is generally classified as thoracic, high lumbar (L1 or L2), midlumbar (L3), low lumbar

Disclosures: The author has nothing to disclose.

[a] Olson Huff Center, Mission Children's Hospital, 11 Vanderbilt Park Drive, Asheville, NC 28803, USA

[b] Department of Pediatrics, CB# 7220, 110E North Medical Drive, University of North Carolina School of Medicine, Chapel Hill, NC 27599-7220, USA

* Olson Huff Center, Mission Children's Hospital, 11 Vanderbilt Park Drive, Asheville, NC 28803.

E-mail address: adsandler@pol.net

Pediatr Clin N Am 57 (2010) 879–892

doi:10.1016/j.pcl.2010.07.009

0031-3955/10/$ – see front matter © 2010 Elsevier Inc. All rights reserved.

pediatric.theclinics.com

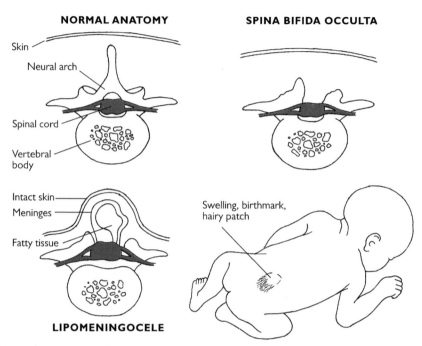

Fig. 1. The spectrum of spina bifida occulta. Abnormalities of this kind are common and usually asymptomatic. (*From* Sandler A. Living with spina bifida: a guide for families and professionals Chapel Hill (NC): University of North Carolina Press; 1997. p. 15; with permission.)

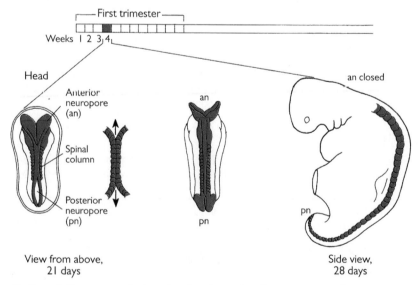

Fig. 2. Neurulation occurs during the fourth week of gestation. The process probably involves several genes important in folate-dependent biosynthesis. (*From* Sandler A. Living with spina bifida: a guide for families and professionals Chapel Hill (NC): University of North Carolina Press; 1997. p. 13; with permission.)

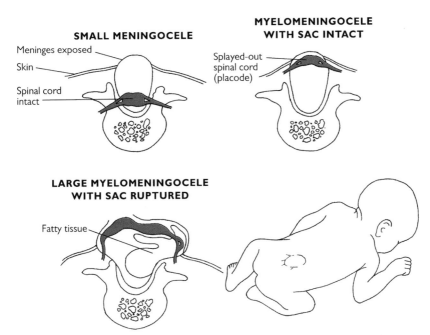

SMALL MENINGOCELE

Meninges exposed

Skin

Spinal cord intact

MYELOMENINGOCELE WITH SAC INTACT

Splayed-out spinal cord (placode)

LARGE MYELOMENINGOCELE WITH SAC RUPTURED

Fatty tissue

Fig. 3. Myelomeningoceles and open spina bifida. Neural elements, including malformed spinal cord, meninges, and fatty tissue are exposed. (*From* Sandler A. Living with spina bifida: a guide for families and professionals Chapel Hill (NC): University of North Carolina Press; 1997. p. 16; with permission.)

(L4 or L5), or sacral. Asymmetry of sensory loss or weakness is common. Most children with low lumbar (L5) or sacral myelomeningocele have absent sensation around the anus, perineum, and feet, but some individuals with lower sacral lesions may have no detectable sensory loss. Children with L1 or L2 lesions may have some hip flexion and adduction but no quadriceps strength to extend the knees. Those with L3 lesions may have knee flexion but paralysis of ankles and feet. Children with L4 and L5 lesions have quadriceps strength (for knee extension) and may have some hamstring (for knee flexion) and anterior tibialis strength (for ankle dorsiflexion). Those with S1 lesions may have functioning glutei (involved in hip extension) and gastrocnemii (involved in ankle plantar flexion). Assessment of motor function is important in predicting mobility and the need for bracing and also serves as useful baseline information in determining whether neurologic deterioration from tethering is occurring.

Functional mobility outcomes for different levels of spina bifida and the need for bracing have been reviewed extensively.[2,3] Children with sacral lesions usually walk by the age of 2 to 3 years and may require bracing at the ankles. Those with L3 paralysis usually require forearm crutches and bracing above the knees. Children with high lumbar or thoracic lesions may eventually stand upright and walk with extensive support of the hips, knees, and ankles. Most children with midlumbar spina bifida, who are able to ambulate with crutches and braces, rely increasingly on wheelchairs for mobility as they get older.

In addition to the disruption of motor and sensory nerves, myelomeningocele affects the sacral parasympathetic nerves that supply the muscular walls of the bladder, urethra, and rectum, and are critically important in sexual functions. Sympathetic nerves controlling the bladder outlet, which originate in the lumbar region of spinal cord, are also typically involved. Bladder and bowel dysfunctions are present in almost all children with myelomeningocele along with varying degrees of sexual dysfunction.

HYDROCEPHALUS AND CHIARI MALFORMATION

Most babies with myelomeningocele have a complex brain malformation, Chiari type II, with associated hydrocephalus.[4–6] Among patients with Chiari II malformations, 80% of those with sacral lesions and more than 90% of those with higher-level lesions receive a shunt. The Chiari II malformation consists of downward displacement of the cerebellum, elongation and upward displacement of the medulla and fourth ventricle, dysgenesis of the corpus callosum, a small posterior fossa, and associated hydrocephalus (Fig. 4). This complex anomaly arises in the fifth week of gestation as a consequence of abnormal neurulation. The Chiari malformation is commonly asymptomatic, but may present with a spectrum of symptoms and signs related to brainstem compression and lower cranial nerve dysfunction. About 30% of infants with myelomeningocele have mild symptoms, including feeding difficulties and gastroesophageal reflux, whereas 5% have more severe symptoms, including stridor, weak cry, failure to thrive, apnea, and cyanosis ("Chiari crisis").

Abnormal CSF dynamics leads to hydrocephalus, which may be present prenatally (the so-called lemon sign on fetal ultrasonography). Neonatal signs include large or rapidly enlarging head circumference, bulging anterior fontanel, and split sagittal suture. Ventriculoperitoneal (V-P) shunts are placed in newborns with myelomeningocele and hydrocephalus, allowing control of CSF pressure and ventricular volumes and prevention of progressive hydrocephalus.

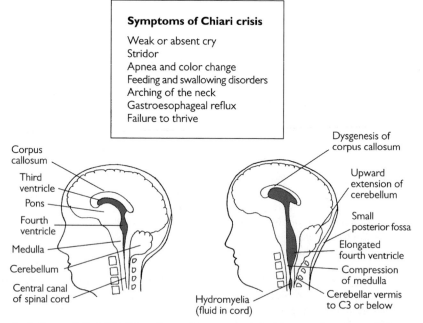

Symptoms of Chiari crisis

Weak or absent cry
Stridor
Apnea and color change
Feeding and swallowing disorders
Arching of the neck
Gastroesophageal reflux
Failure to thrive

Fig. 4. Features of the Chiari II malformation, compared with normal anatomy (*left panel*). Symptoms of Chiari crisis may occur in infancy because of brainstem compression. (*From* Sandler A. Living with spina bifida: a guide for families and professionals Chapel Hill (NC): University of North Carolina Press; 1997. p. 68; with permission.)

ASSOCIATED NEUROLOGIC DISORDERS

Approximately 15% to 20% of children with spina bifida have seizures in childhood.[7] Seizures are more likely in children with shunts, especially in those with previous shunt infections, and the onset of a seizure may indicate a shunt malfunction. The seizures are usually generalized tonic-clonic type and respond well to antiepileptic medications.

Oculomotor disorders, such as difficulty with visual tracking, are common in spina bifida and may be related to the effects of Chiari malformation and hydrocephalus on midbrain gaze centers. Strabismus occurs in 20% of the patients and may require surgery. Even in the absence of hydrocephalus and Chiari malformation, fine motor function may be impaired, probably because of cerebellar and cervical cord abnormalities.[8]

Parents and clinicians need to remain vigilant for signs of neurologic deterioration in children with spina bifida. The signs of shunt failure (rapidly enlarging head circumference, swelling or redness along the shunt track) are usually clear in the infant and toddler. In young children, shunt failure may present acutely with headache, irritability, lethargy, and vomiting, but signs of shunt malfunction may be subtle and insidious, including mild drowsiness and impaired attention and coordination. Chiari II malformation or cervical hydromyelia may present with neck pain, progressive spasticity, or ataxia.

Another important cause of neurologic deterioration is tethered cord.[9] During normal growth, the spinal cord ascends within the canal so that the conus moves from L4 to L2 between birth and puberty. In spina bifida, the abnormal cord may be tethered to the scar tissue or bony deformities, leading to ischemic damage. Associated spinal cord anomalies such as hydromyelia and cord lipomas may also cause neurologic problems. Clinical signs are most common around the age of 6 to 12 years, including deterioration of walking, back pain, leg pain, spasticity, increasing scoliosis, progressive foot deformity, and deterioration in bladder and bowel function. Progressive weakness over time on manual muscle testing and changes in bladder function are key clinical findings. The back pain is typically worsened with activity and relieved by rest. Tethering is generally diagnosed on clinical grounds, although magnetic resonance imaging of the spine, urodynamics, and electrophysiologic testing may provide additional data. Surgical release of the tethered cord effectively relieves pain and may arrest neurologic deterioration.[10]

ORTHOPEDIC IMPAIRMENTS

Muscle weakness leads to abnormal positioning in utero. Consequently, 50% of the babies with myelomeningocele have significant foot deformity at birth ("clubfoot"), including calcaneovalgus, equinovarus, and vertical talus (**Fig. 5**). During early childhood, further deformity may occur from ongoing muscle imbalance, postural effects of gravity, and growth. A plantigrade foot in neutral position is essential for optimal walking, and a well-positioned foot may protect against skin breakdown. Hence physical therapy, casting, subcutaneous releases, and postoperative splinting are commonly needed in infancy. More definitive surgical reconstruction, including releases, tendon transfers, and bony surgery, may be required at the age of around 12 to 24 months, and bracing is usually required to maintain alignment and improve mobility.[11]

Hip flexors and adductors are innervated by L1 and L2, whereas hip extensors and abductors are innervated by L5 and S1. Hence, muscle imbalance and hip instability are common in spina bifida. Subluxed or dislocated hips occur in 25% to 50% of

Calcaneovalgus

Equinovarus

Vertical talus

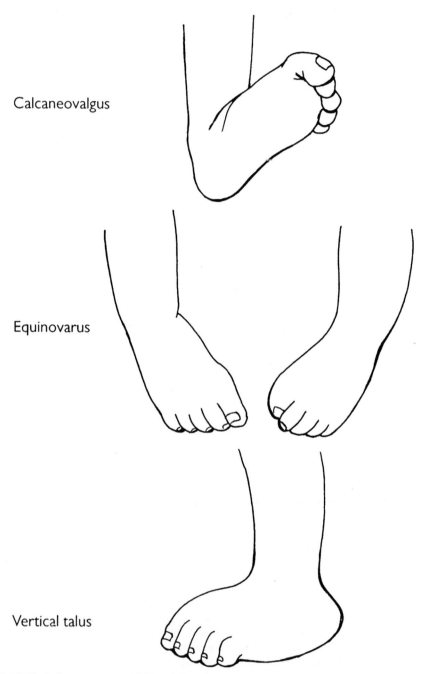

Fig. 5. Typical appearances of foot deformities in spina bifida, including calcaneovalgus, equinovarus, and vertical talus. (*From* Sandler A. Living with spina bifida: a guide for families and professionals Chapel Hill (NC): University of North Carolina Press; 1997. p. 137; with permission.)

newborns with high or midlumbar lesions, and another 25% become unstable during early childhood. The main concern is not the effects on walking but that asymmetric hips and associated pelvic obliquity may cause scoliosis, seating problems, and pressure sores.

Scoliosis may be congenital or acquired. Congenital scoliosis occurs in 15% to 25% of newborns with spina bifida, most commonly with thoracic lesions. Acquired (or "paralytic") scoliosis is usually first noted in early school age, and the condition may progress rapidly, especially during puberty. Tethering and hydromyelia, pelvic obliquity, and asymmetric motor function may cause progressive scoliosis. Severe kyphosis may be present at birth, most commonly associated with lumbar myelomeningoceles, posing a challenge to the surgeons performing the primary closure. Severe scoliosis and kyphosis may interfere with sitting and walking, and may compromise respiratory function. Lightweight molded orthoses may prevent progression and/or delay the need for spinal fusion and stabilization with rods.

BLADDER AND BOWEL DYSFUNCTION

Myelomeningocele is almost always associated with neurogenic bladder.[12] Despite normal urinary tracts in 90% of the children on ultrasonography, 1 in 3 newborns has a "hostile bladder" and is at risk for developing hydronephrosis and renal scarring. Urodynamics (also known as video urodynamic studies) is valuable in the diagnosis of bladder dysfunction, detecting those with hostile features, such as high bladder pressures and outlet resistance (detrusor-sphincter dyssynergia). Clean intermittent catheterization (CIC) and anticholinergics, or vesicostomy, may be needed in the neonatal period to prevent renal complications. Monitoring the urinary tract with ultrasonography every 6 to 12 months is important to detect pelvicaliectasis or hydronephrosis. Also, catheterized urine samples are important to detect bacteriuria, and a voiding cystourethrogram may be needed to rule out vesicoureteral reflux. The incomplete emptying of a neurogenic bladder predisposes to bacteriuria, but this condition is usually asymptomatic and does not require treatment. However, in the presence of high bladder pressures and/or vesicoureteral reflux, the kidneys are at risk for pyelonephritis. Hence, babies with reflux should be on prophylactic antibiotics and CIC.

Children with neurogenic bladder are unable to perceive bladder fullness and lack coordination between detrusor contraction and sphincter relaxation. For some, this lack of coordination poses a risk to their kidneys, but for all it presents a challenge of continence. Lapides and colleagues[13] revolutionized the management of spina bifida with the advent of CIC. Detailed accounts of the techniques are available elsewhere.[2] In addition to CIC, pharmacologic management includes the use of anticholinergic medications to inhibit detrusor contractions and increase storage volumes. With CIC 4 or 5 times daily, anticholinergic medications, and good clinical care, 70% to 90% of children are reliably dry or have only occasional episodes of wetting. Some children with very small capacity bladders may require surgical augmentation with the cecum (enterocystoplasty). One variation is the Mitrofanoff procedure, in which the appendix is used to connect the augmented bladder to the abdominal wall at or near the umbilicus and the continence ostomy is then used for CIC.

Most children with spina bifida have a neurogenic bowel, developing constipation because of decreased bowel motility. Efforts to control constipation in early childhood can help to prevent urinary tract infections. Initiation of a bowel program by the age of 3 to 5 years with regular assisted evacuation of stool is an important habilitation goal. The social acceptance of the young child at school entry is enhanced by having predictable bowel movements and few episodes of incontinence. The choice of bowel management methods should be based on individualized assessment and include education to enhance the family's motivation and treatment adherence.[14] Methods for bowel management include habit training, digital stimulation, suppository or mini-enema daily (or every other day), cone enema (with colostomy irrigation kit), and Malone antegrade continence enema (ACE). The ACE has become accepted as an important salvage procedure for intractable constipation and fecal incontinence.[15]

COGNITIVE IMPAIRMENTS

Individuals with spina bifida frequently have below-average cognitive abilities, and mild intellectual disability is not uncommon.[16] Abstract reasoning, visual perceptual abilities, and visual motor integration are typically weak. Verbal reasoning score tends to be higher than that for nonverbal reasoning. Higher-level lesions are associated with lower IQ, although this association does not have predictive usefulness. The presence of hydrocephalus is not in itself a major risk factor for intellectual development. Indeed, many children with myelomeningocele and without hydrocephalus have a neuropsychological profile similar to those with hydrocephalus. Among those with hydrocephalus and shunts, ventriculitis and other major shunt complications may lead to acquired brain injury and more severe intellectual disability. Attention, organization, and executive functions may be impaired, and many children may meet the criteria for attention-deficit/hyperactivity disorder. Children of school age may show relative strengths in social skills, expressive language, reading, and spelling. Problem solving, writing, and math skills are typical areas of weakness.[17]

The combination of paralysis and cognitive impairments are major challenges to the development of independent living skills. Doting parents and other family members can unwittingly behave in ways that encourage dependency. An important goal of habilitation is for the child with spina bifida to assist in self-care and to participate in activities of daily living. Young children should be encouraged to assist in diaper changes, putting on braces, bathing, dressing, and catheterization. Beginning this process early helps to prevent learned helplessness, dependency, and severe impairments in adaptive function.

SKIN PROBLEMS

The most common cause of skin injury is pressure from prolonged sitting in one position. Persistent redness over the ischial tuberosity may progress to blistering and skin breakdown. Pressure sores can be extraordinarily slow to heal, and exact an enormous cost both in health care expenditures and in loss of function. Other common injuries include burns and trauma to insensate feet, emphasizing the importance of health education and anticipatory guidance in prevention of secondary disability.

OTHER PEDIATRIC HEALTH ISSUES

The motor paralysis of spina bifida leads to decreased caloric expenditure and obesity in at least 20% of school-aged children. Obesity may seriously compromise mobility and pose additional challenges to optimal health and habilitation. Changes in body mass index and skin fold thickness are useful indicators of obesity in the clinic. Nutrition education, motivational interviewing, and family-based support may help to prevent obesity.

Short stature is common in spina bifida, affecting 80% of those with lesions at or above L3. Small lower limbs, spinal deformities, and scoliosis may contribute, but differences in frequency and amplitude of growth hormone secretion have been reported. Other neurosecretory abnormalities have been implicated in the development of precocious puberty in children with spina bifida and hydrocephalus. Referral to a pediatric endocrinologist may be needed for control of rapidly progressing puberty with leuprolide acetate (luteinizing hormone receptor inhibitor).

After a report of a cluster of cases of intraoperative anaphylaxis in children with spina bifida in 1989, it was estimated that 18% to 40% had latex allergy. Latex allergy is more common in children with a history of allergies and asthma and in those who have had multiple operations. The Nursing Council of the Spina Bifida Association has spearheaded efforts worldwide to raise awareness of latex allergy and institute latex precautions for primary and secondary prevention, thereby decreasing morbidity and mortality from this common complication.[18]

THE HISTORY OF CARE OF THE CHILD WITH SPINA BIFIDA

The history of health care of children with spina bifida has included several revolutionary and dramatic advances. In 1956, engineer John Holter's only son Casey was born with a myelomeningocele. Holter's efforts to save his son's life led to the development of the Spitz-Holter valve and other effective shunt valves.[19] In the 1960s, ventriculoatrial shunting was commonly done, but V-P shunting soon became the standard treatment (**Fig. 6**). Although much progress has been made in the prevention of ventriculitis, there continues to be a high incidence of unpredictable shunt failure. In the past 10 years, alternative techniques for treating hydrocephalus have been available, including the endoscopic third ventriculostomy.[20,21]

In 1972, Lapides and colleagues[13] revolutionized the management of spina bifida using CIC. This simple procedure allowed complete bladder emptying, thereby protecting the kidneys from infection and preventing or reversing hydronephrosis. This technique remains the mainstay of urological management of the neurogenic bladder and has prevented countless deaths from renal failure.

Before the 1960s, most newborns with spina bifida in the United States and United Kingdom were not treated surgically because the prognosis was thought to be poor. In 1971, Lorber[22] and other investigators published criteria based on prognostic factors for selecting which infants to treat and which to allow to die. Until the early 1980s, many nurseries used these criteria to select infants for treatment or nontreatment, although some centers, most notably the Children's Memorial Hospital in Chicago, questioned the appropriateness of selection and published large series on consecutive nonselected patients with myelomeningocele.[5] Based on the birth of a girl (Baby Jane Doe) with spina bifida and hydrocephalus in 1983, whose parents declined surgery, the US Congress adopted Baby Doe rules as amendments to the Child Abuse and Neglect Funding Requirements for the United States, mandating the provision of life-sustaining medical treatment to seriously ill infants. Since then almost all newborns with spina bifida in the United States have been treated.

In 1970, Hide and Semple[23] described a comprehensive multidisciplinary outpatient clinic in Oxford, England, attended by a pediatrician, orthopedic surgeon, pediatric surgeon, urologist, physical therapist, nurse, and social worker. Similar spina bifida clinics were developed in the United States and were functional in almost every state during the 1980s and 1990s. During the past 10 to 15 years it appears that financial pressures, and perhaps declining prevalence of spina bifida, have affected outpatient programs for children with spina bifida, affecting the participation of some specialists and the extent of care coordination.

In 1972, Brock and Sutcliffe[24] reported the association between increased amniotic α-fetoprotein (AFP) and NTDs. This knowledge opened the door to maternal

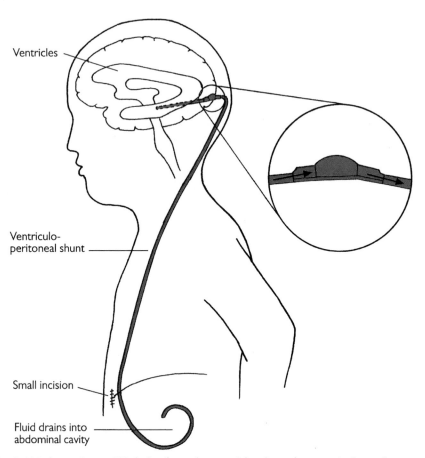

Ventricles

Ventriculo-
peritoneal shunt

Small incision

Fluid drains into
abdominal cavity

Fig. 6. V-P shunt. Excess CSF drains from the ventricles through a ventricular catheter and pressure-sensitive valve into the peritoneal space. (*From* Sandler A. Living with spina bifida: a guide for families and professionals Chapel Hill (NC): University of North Carolina Press; 1997. p. 66; with permission.)

serum AFP screening between 15 and 20 weeks of gestation. Comprehensive screening programs that include counseling, AFP screening, high-resolution ultrasonography, and amniocentesis have been an important breakthrough in the management of NTDs.

In 1981, the first attempts to surgically treat hydrocephalus in the human fetus were reported, but subsequent case series showed an unacceptably high rate of morbidity and mortality. In 1997, in utero repair of myelomeningocele via hysterotomy began, based on animal models and evidence that neurologic function deteriorates during gestation.[25] By 2003, 234 women had fetal repair of myelomeningocele, and preliminary evidence showed that only 49% of infants had a shunt placed by the age of 1 year.[26] The Management of Myelomeningocele Study (MOMS) is a randomized trial of prenatal versus postnatal myelomeningocele repair funded by the National Institute of Child Health and Human Development, which is nearing completion at 3 clinical centers. The trial has 2 primary end points: the need for shunting by 12 months and neurodevelopmental outcome (Bayley scores and functional motor level) at 30 months. To date, more than 150 of the planned enrollment of 200 subjects have been randomized, and it remains to be seen whether prenatal surgery represents another breakthrough in the treatment of spina bifida.

ETIOLOGY OF NTDS: RECENT ADVANCES

Folates are cofactors for one-carbon transfer reactions that are important in the biosynthesis of methionine and proteins. Deficiency in 5,10-methylene tetrahydrofolate reductase, an enzyme important in the conversion of homocysteine to methionine, is a risk factor for NTDs. Folate deficiency is associated with elevated homocysteine levels and is also a risk factor for NTDs. Numerous mutant mouse models attest to the ease of disruption of neurulation due to genetic variants, and recent evidence implicates a variety of genetic variants in folate and vitamin B_{12} metabolism that may affect risk for NTDs.[27] Other factors associated with NTDs include chromosomal disorders, maternal exposure to valproic acid, hyperthermia during early pregnancy, and maternal diabetes.

FOLIC ACID AND PREVENTION OF NTDS

The 1991 United Kingdom Medical Research Council trial showed that 4 mg of folic acid around conception and in early pregnancy reduced recurrence risk among women with previous NTD-affected pregnancy from 3.5% to 1%.[28] Several subsequent trials have demonstrated that supplementation with folic acid reduced the risk of NTDs in the general population by 50% to 70%.[29–31]

Natural food folates have poor bioavailability and stability, so prevention efforts have focused on periconceptional supplementation and fortification of foods. Mandatory folic acid fortification of enriched grain products marketed in the United States since 1998 has been associated with an important decline in prevalence of NTDs of between 35% and 78%, or approximately 1000 fewer NTD-affected pregnancies per year.[32] Brent and Oakley[33] and other researchers have argued that folic acid fortification levels are too low and that prevention efforts could be more effective in the United States and elsewhere. To date, there are no proven adverse effects of folic acid fortification. There is debate on the extent to which folic acid–preventable NTDs are being prevented and whether racial/ethnic variation in prevalence is due to underlying ethnic differences in susceptibility or differences in case ascertainment.[27,34] One of the major challenges in primary prevention of spina bifida is how to reach Latin American women, who have higher risk of NTDs and lower folic acid intakes than non-Latin American women. Current public health strategies include adding folic acid to corn masa flour.

EVIDENCE-BASED PRACTICE IN SPINA BIFIDA: CURRENT CHALLENGES IN QUALITY CARE

It is hardly surprising that such a complex and multisystem birth defect continues to challenge clinicians in their efforts to provide evidence-based answers to important clinical questions and dilemmas. In 2003, the National Institutes of Health, Centers of Disease Control and Prevention, Spina Bifida Association, and others sponsored a multidisciplinary symposium to highlight key questions and priorities for further clinical research.[35] A few clinical questions highlighted at that symposium are listed to illustrate the scope of the challenge and opportunity for further important research:

- What is the optimal treatment of hydrocephalus?
- What is the best method for evaluating and monitoring shunt function?

- Which patients would benefit most from tethered cord release?
- What is the optimal management of hip dislocation?
- How to prevent and manage osteoporosis?
- How can animal models be developed to explore neuromodulation of bladder function?
- What is the optimal management of reproductive issues in women with spina bifida?
- What are the pathophysiologic factors that affect skin breakdown?
- What are the instructional and developmental interventions that facilitate learning?
- How best to promote optimal psychosexual development and sexual adaptation?
- How to effectively teach and promote self-care?

Further advances in spina bifida health care will require a commitment to outcomes-based clinical research and would be greatly facilitated by translational research, multicenter trials, and development of a registry. This need is illustrated by the following 3 cutting-edge areas of clinical research: management of hydrocephalus, innovative approaches to enhance bladder function, and transition to adult health care.

Approximately 40% of new shunts fail within a year, and 80% within 10 years. It is troubling that outcomes of treatment of hydrocephalus have changed little in recent decades despite advances in shunt technology. This lack of improvement has led to a renewed focus in neurosurgery on understanding the pathophysiology of hydrocephalus and developing more effective treatment for this condition.

DISCUSSION OF CONSERVATIVE SHUNT PLACEMENT (THE CHICAGO EXPERIENCE)

Another new area of research is the procedure described by Xiao and colleagues[36] for rerouting functioning lumbar motor nerves to sacral root motor neurons in an effort to innervate the lower urinary tract. Several children who have undergone this procedure in recent years have been able to initiate a reflex bladder contraction by scratching or rubbing the ipsilateral sensory dermatome, but questions about effectiveness and concerns about transient weakness remain unresolved.

Transition to adult health care remains a major challenge. Much of the progress in management of spina bifida has come from the pooled experience of comprehensive multidisciplinary clinics in pediatric settings. Young adults leaving these pediatric settings struggle to find continuing sources of health care. The burdens are especially acute because of the lack of care coordination and insurance coverage in this age group.

A FUNCTIONAL HOLISTIC DEVELOPMENTAL PERSPECTIVE

This article summarizes some of the key clinical issues in the care of children with this complex birth defect. The need for a coordinated approach among clinicians of different subspecialties is clear. In addition to the core pediatric surgical specialists (neurosurgeons, orthopedic surgeons, and urologists), nursing and allied health professionals (including physical therapists, occupational therapists, and psychologists) help to enhance family education and the child's functional outcomes. A pediatric developmental perspective emphasizes a child's growth and changing capacities, assessing a child's strengths and weaknesses and helping to anticipate challenges and opportunities. Optimal management of the whole child with spina bifida involves more than the sum of the subspecialty care of his or her parts. Instead, it calls for a flexible and dynamic partnership between the clinicians, the parents, and the child; one that continually strives to enhance health, self-care, learning, and participation in activities and ultimately secures a life of quality.

REFERENCES

1. Van Allen MI, Kalousek DK, Chernoff GF, et al. Evidence for multi-site closure of the neural tube in humans. Am J Med Genet 1993;47:723–43.
2. Sandler A. In living with spina bifida. Chapel Hill (NC): UNC Press; 2004. p. 84, 95, 159–67.
3. Mazur JM, Kyle S. Efficacy of bracing the lower limbs and ambulation training in children with myelomeningocele. Dev Med Child Neurol 2004;46:352–6.
4. McLone DG, Knepper PA. The cause of Chiari II malformation: a unified theory. Pediatr Neurosci 1989;15:1–12.
5. McLone DG. Continuing concepts in the management of spina bifida. Pediatr Neurosurg 1992;18:254–6.
6. Rauzzino M, Oakes WJ. Chiari II malformation and syringomyelia. Neurosurg Clin N Am 1995;6:293–309.
7. Liptak GS. Neural tube defects. In: Batshaw ML, editor. Children with disabilities. 4th edition. Baltimore (MD): Paul H Brookes; 1997. p. 529–52.
8. Muen WJ, Bannister CM. Hand function in subjects with spina bifida. Eur J Pediatr Surg 1997;7(Suppl 1):18–22.
9. Liptak GS. Tethered spinal cord: update of an analysis of published articles. Eur J Pediatr Surg 1996;5:21–3.
10. Schoenmakers MA, Gooskens RH, Gulmans VA, et al. Long-term outcome of neurosurgical untethering on neurosegmental motor and ambulation levels. Dev Med Child Neurol 2003;45:551–5.
11. Swank M, Dias L. Myelomeningocele: a review of the orthopedic aspects of 206 patients treated from birth with no selection criteria. Dev Med Child Neurol 1992; 34:1047–52.
12. Anderson PA, Travers AH. Development of hydronephrosis in spina bifida patients: predictive factors and management. Br J Urol 1993;72:958–61.
13. Lapides J, Diokno AC, Silber SJ, et al. Clean, intermittent self-catheterization in the treatment of urinary tract disease. J Urol 1972;107:458–61.
14. Leibold S. Neurogenic bowel and continence programs for the individual with spina bifida. J Pediatr Rehabil Med 2008;1:325–36.
15. Hensle TW, Reiley EA, Chang DT. The Malone antegrade continence enema procedure in the management of patients with spina bifida. J Am Coll Surg 1998;186:669–74.
16. Friedrich WN, Lovejoy MC, Shaffer J, et al. Cognitive abilities and achievement status of children with myelomeningocele: a contemporary sample. J Pediatr Psychol 1991;16:423–8.
17. Barf HA, Verhoef M, Jennekens-Schinkel A, et al. Cognitive status of young adults with spina bifida. Dev Med Child Neurol 2003;45:813–20.
18. Grayhack JJ, Meeropol E. Latex allergy. In: Sarwack JF, Lubicky JP, editors. Caring for the child with spina bifida. Amer Acad Orthoped Surgeons; 2002. p. 493–501.
19. Boockvar JA, Loudon W, Sutton LN. Development of the Spitz-Holter valve in Philadelphia. J Neurosurg 2001;95:145–7.

20. Teo C, Jones R. Management of hydrocephalus by endoscopic third ventriculostomy in patients with myelomeningocele. Pediatr Neurosurg 1996;25:57–63.
21. Warf BC, Campbell JW. Combined endoscopic third ventriculostomy and choroid plexus cauterization as primary treatment of hydrocephalus for infants with myelomeningocele: long-term results of a prospective intent-to-treat study in 115 East African infants. J Neurosurg Pediatr 2008;2:310–6.
22. Lorber J. Results of treatment of myelomeningocele. An analysis of 524 unselected cases, with special reference to possible selection for treatment. Dev Med Child Neurol 1971;13:279–303.
23. Hide DW, Semple C. Coordinated care of the child with spina bifida. Lancet 1970; 2:603–4.
24. Brock DJH, Sutcliffe RG. Alpha-fetoprotein in the antenatal diagnosis of anencephaly and spina bifida. Lancet 1972;2:197–9.
25. Bruner JP, Tulipan N, Paschall RL, et al. Fetal surgery for myelomeningocele and the incidence of shunt-dependent hydrocephalus. JAMA 1999;282:1819–25.
26. Danzer E, Finkel RS, Rintoul NE, et al. Reversal of hindbrain herniation after maternal-fetal surgery for myelomeningocele subsequently impacts on brain stem function. Neuropediatrics 2008;39:359–62.
27. Molloy AM, Kirke PN, Troendle JF, et al. Maternal vitamin B12 status and risk of neural tube defects in a population with high neural tube defect prevalence and no folic acid fortification. Pediatrics 2009;123:917–23.
28. Prevention of neural tube defects: results of the Medical Research Council vitamin study. MRC Vitamin Study Research Group. Lancet 1991;338:131–7.
29. Czeizl AE, Dudas I. Prevention of first occurrence of neural tube defects by periconceptional vitamin supplementation. N Engl J Med 1992;327:1832–5.
30. Werler MM, Shapiro S, Mitchell AA. Periconceptional folic acid exposure and risk of occurrent neural tube defects. JAMA 1993;269:1257–61.
31. Berry RJ, Li Z, Erickson JD, et al. Prevention of neural-tube defects with folic acid in China. China-US Collaborative Projects for Neural Tube Prevention. N Engl J Med 1999;341:1485–90.
32. Williams LJ, Rasmussen SA, Flores A, et al. Decline in prevalence of spina bifida and anencephaly by race/ethnicity. Pediatrics 2005;116:580–6.
33. Brent RL, Oakley GP. The folate debate. Pediatrics 2006;117:1418–9.
34. Rader JI, Schneeman BO. Prevalence of neural tube defects, folate status, and folate fortification of enriched cereal-grain products in the United States. Pediatrics 2006;117:1394–9.
35. Liptak GS, editor. Evidence-based practice in spina bifida: developing a research agenda. Washington, DC: Spina Bifida Association of America; 2003.
36. Xiao CG, Du MX, Li B, et al. An artificial somatic-autonomic reflex pathway procedure for bladder control in children with spina bifida. J Urol 2005;173:2112–6.

Need for the Life Course Model for Spina Bifida

Mark E. Swanson, MD, MPH

KEYWORDS

• Spina bifida • Transition • Self-management • ICF

In previous generations, people with conditions such as spina bifida (SB), sickle cell disease, cystic fibrosis, and muscular dystrophy were not expected to live very far, if at all, into adulthood. If these people did live, health care professionals and other providers were pleased that they had even lived that long. Because children with chronic conditions have grown up into adults in increasing numbers,[1–4] they and their families have increasingly questioned whether they have reached their full potential and maximized their participation in adult activities. When standards of care and relevant outcomes are expressed in traditional medical parameters (mortality, morbidity, occurrence of secondary health conditions involving other organ systems), scant attention was paid to the functional outcomes that are the norm for typical young adults, including whether the young adult had a job or sufficient self-directed income, had friendships and relationships, lived independently, and engaged in recreation and other health-promoting activities. Expectations were often low to nonexistent about this group's potential to function well in these domains of adulthood.

Pediatric chronic disease specialists are increasingly recognizing the shortcomings in the quality of life of their patients as they reach adulthood. As patients leave pediatric care, their doctors are moving beyond the issue of a simple transfer of health care to adult doctors to feeling a responsibility and an interest in functional outcomes, in terms of full participation in adult living.[5]

The disability movement of the 1990s, reinforced by the Americans with Disabilities Act and other legislations and policies, has empowered people with disabilities to view themselves differently. These people now aspire to the full quality of life as demonstrated by their typical peers and portrayed in the media. With aspirations, comes an expectation that the systems of services and support will prepare them for these enhanced adult roles.[6]

The findings and conclusions in this article are those of the author and do not necessarily represent the official position of the Centers for Disease Control and Prevention.
Division of Human Development and Disability, National Center on Birth Defects and Developmental Disabilities, Centers for Disease Control and Prevention, Atlanta, GA, USA
E-mail address: cfu9@cdc.gov

Pediatr Clin N Am 57 (2010) 893–901
doi:10.1016/j.pcl.2010.08.001
0031-3955/10/$ – see front matter © 2010 Elsevier Inc. All rights reserved.

TRANSFER OF HEALTH SERVICES

Because of the lack of adult health care providers with expertise in SB, many young people struggle to find health services. Many patients stay with their pediatric provider well into their adulthood, reflecting the trend seen in other childhood-onset lifelong conditions. Indeed, Boston Children's Hospital now allows patients up to 35 years of age to attend certain clinics run by their pediatric staff. Still, as children with SB reach adulthood, most of them lose access to health care providers who have knowledge about SB. This situation places an increasing responsibility on the patients to understand their own condition, the pattern of symptoms unique to them, the self-management of symptoms that works, and the threshold for seeking medical attention.[7] Shunt function typifies this situation. Young adult patients have a long experience with possibly shunt-related symptoms, such as headache and fever. Ideally, these patients would be able to make measured decisions on what intensity and duration of symptoms can be self-managed and when to seek care for possible shunt malfunction. Management of urinary symptoms is a similar situation. This enhanced self-management would be desirable if the patient has access to experienced adult health care providers but is even more critical when the access is limited. Covering these eventualities requires preparation of the young patient with SB, starting in early childhood.

The Life Course Model merges several concepts and principles related to children with disabilities and provides a framework for services and research to achieve the desired adult outcomes (**Fig. 1**).

NORMAL CHILD DEVELOPMENT

Children are dynamic in their progress from infancy to adulthood. Their development follows a series of predictable stages or milestones in each of their domains of development. An important principle is that stages in development generally have to follow a sequence, that is, important stages cannot be skipped to move on to future stages. One cannot walk until one learns to stand upright. This principle applies to motor milestones as well as language, cognitive, emotional, and behavioral milestones. The sequence of development may be tighter and more predictable in the preschool years but still needs to be followed in school years and adolescence.[8]

If a critical milestone is missed, it may be difficult to go back and relearn that stage. For instance, children who fail to resolve their struggle for autonomy at ages 2 to 3 years may struggle with autonomy in their teen years and may possibly have trouble with authority and self-control throughout their lives.

INTERNATIONAL CLASSIFICATION OF FUNCTIONING, DISABILITY AND HEALTH

The International Classification of Functioning, Disability and Health (ICF)[9] was developed as the latest addition to the family of international classification systems. Thinking that the previous International Classification of Diseases codes were heavily medical and deficit-oriented, experts proposed a new system of classification oriented to function and participation rather than disease and limitations. The ICF, proposed in 1992 and finalized in 2001, is based on the principles that (1) activities and participation are the desired outcomes that should be monitored and measured and (2) these outcomes are determined by an interaction between impairments (of a body part or system) and other factors (environmental and personal). These principles suggest that a responsive accommodative environment will lead to a higher degree of function and participation than a less accommodating environment. Environment

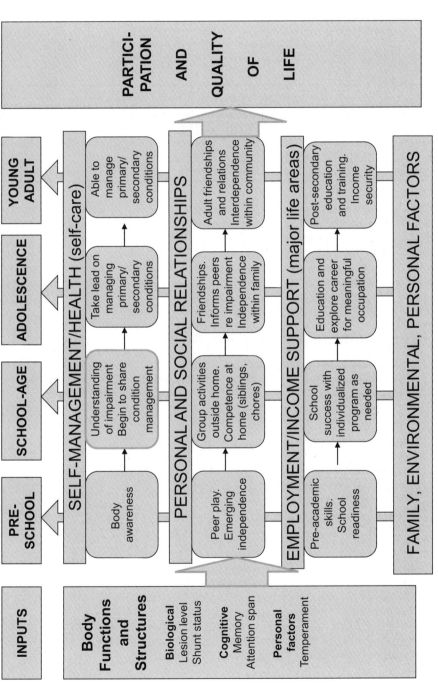

Fig. 1. The life course model for SB.

includes family, community, school, and service systems and encompasses attitudes as well as direct services. Although the details used in the ICF to measure environmental factors and participation outcomes can be cumbersome, the ICF is especially useful in its broad categorization of outcomes, specifically its participation domains or categories. The ICF is a world-recognized classification system that now shapes almost all current discussions of disability-related services and science.

ICF	System for Classifying Impairments, Activities, and Participation
Impairment	Affected body structure or function (eg, SB, paralysis, cognitive limitation, primary emotional disturbance, sickle cell disease)
Activity	Execution of a task or action by an individual (often in a controlled situation, such as home)
Participation	Involvement in a life situation (or performing activities in the real world)

What is most appealing about the ICF in relation to SB is the recognition that a biosocial model is needed to explain the differences in outcomes for persons with SB. A biologic model would suggest that the initial lesion and birth anatomy would greatly determine the outcomes in children with SB. This suggestion may hold true for some of the biologic outcomes (motor function, cognition) that are heavily influenced by lesion level, anatomic brain differences, and shunt malfunctions, which are always followed in a medical setting.

But the differences in functional outcomes of employment, relationships, and emotional well-being are not explained by these biologic inputs. Other factors must be identified to explain the variation in functional outcomes. So the ICF offers 2 concepts:

- Participation is the desired outcome.
- Participation results from an interaction between the impairment and environmental response.

There are 8 areas of participation defined by the ICF:

1. Interpersonal interactions and relationships
2. Major life areas
3. Self-care (management)
4. Learning and applying knowledge
5. Communication
6. Domestic life
7. Community, social, and civic life
8. General tasks and demands.

The authors' Transition Working Group focused on adaptations of the first 3 areas of participation in creating the Life Course Model. These areas were thought to be most compatible with a participation theme and a developmental model that would track progress from early childhood to adulthood.

The authors have operationalized the ICF to define optimal adult function as successful participation in the first 3 areas. Certain elements of the unchosen 5 areas were incorporated into the 3 themes chosen for this project.

Definitions

Interpersonal interactions and relationships[9]:
Informal social relationships

Entering into relationships with others, such as casual relationships with people living in the same community or residence; with coworkers, students, playmates; or with people from similar backgrounds or professions.

Formal relationships

Creating and maintaining specific relationships in formal settings, such as with employers, professionals, or service providers.

Intimate relationships

Creating and maintaining close or romantic relationships between individuals, such as husband and wife, lovers, or sexual partners.

Major life areas[9]

Education

Work

Economic life

Self-care[9]

Looking after one's health

Ensuring physical comfort, health, and physical and mental well-being by maintaining a balanced diet and an appropriate level of physical activity, keeping warm or cool, avoiding harms to health, following safe sex practices, including using condoms, and getting immunizations and regular physical examinations.

Toileting

Planning and performing the elimination of human waste (menstruation, urination, and defecation), and cleaning oneself afterwards.

Impairments are the underlying conditions that are inputs into the Life Course Model. People with impairments are not unhealthy or limited in participation. The goal of persons with impairments should be assumed to be the same as for those who are nonimpaired, namely full participation.

INTEGRATION OF THE ICF AND DEVELOPMENTAL APPROACH ASSUMPTIONS/VALUES

1. Children with disabilities and their families have the same aspirations (ICF domains) for successful adult living as those without disabilities.
2. Successful adult living follows effective preparation, which is demonstrated by making steady progress in life domains, starting in the early childhood.
3. Impairment and its subsequent interventions (treatment) and environmental response can adversely affect the trajectory of development in children with chronic health conditions, such as SB, and lead to disability when environmental factors are insufficiently accommodative to allow participation.
4. The natural history of many impairments is unknown for 2 reasons:
   - Only recently have children lived well into adulthood.
   - Physical health and, especially, functional outcomes have not been documented.
5. Lack of knowledgeable adult medical providers and longitudinal data about natural history places more responsibility on individuals and their family for self-care of the impairment.

Because child development is a naturally dynamic process, it is subject to environmental factors that can interrupt the process. Even in children with no body impairment, environmental factors such as a chaotic home, overly critical or lax parenting, unresponsive teachers, unstructured classrooms or dangerous communities can threaten development. Typical children tend to have a greater reserve and capacity to deal with these environmental challenges than a child with a constant impairment.[10] The ability to adjust or accommodate to an environmental stressor is less with a cognitive, motor, or emotional impairment. Critical developmental milestones may be delayed or missed between a permanent impairment and an intermittently unsupportive environment.

By systematically measuring development (proximal outcomes) in children who are at risk for altered development, parents and clinicians can track progress in life domains.[11–13] If a child begins to fall off the normal trajectory in a given domain, there is an opportunity to intervene and bolster progress in that track.

SELF-MANAGEMENT OF CHRONIC ILLNESS

The chronic care model exemplifies many of the principles of self-management of chronic illness. Patients and their families, in essence, are the primary caregivers in chronic illness. Self-management has the goals of promoting health and preventing complications. These goals are accomplished through monitoring of physical and emotional statuses and making appropriate decisions based on self-monitoring.[14] The added benefit to this process is empowerment. Positive results reinforce the process. Self-management includes how to develop and maintain exercise and nutrition programs, manage symptoms, determine when to seek medical help, work effectively with doctors, properly use medications and minimize side effects, find community resources, and discuss the illness with family and friends.

Young people with SB face the challenge of living with a chronic condition that affects multiple organ systems and can require immediate, if not emergency, attention. Because most people have ventricular shunts, they have to monitor symptoms that could be related to shunt malfunction, such as headache, malaise, fever, and weakness. Urinary symptoms have to be interpreted in the light of decreased sensation. Pressure sores also need visual diligence to augment limited sensation. Lower extremity function is dealt with in the face of motor and sensory deficits.

The combination of chronic and acute symptoms places considerable responsibility on the family when the child is young. With independence as an adult goal, a family's health monitoring needs to be a shared responsibility during childhood, with the child steadily taking on more and more of the responsibility for self-management of his or her health.[7] Collaborative management with health care professionals is desirable. Such management is more often available for children with SB because they have access to pediatricians and pediatric-oriented specialists health care professionals who have knowledge of SB and are aware of the key role played by families in providing care.

Management includes the self-care taken on by all children and also the special features of SB. All children learn to manage their own acute symptoms (pain, malaise, fever) and make decisions on when to seek help (from parents or the health care provider). Monitoring of the development of this self-care skill is especially important for children with SB, given the projected need to manage their own health in adulthood and to educate adult health care providers about management of the secondary conditions associated with SB. The chronic care model offers useful guidance for the life course model. Although originally targeted for chronic disease management in adults, the chronic care model offers useful principles and techniques that can be adapted for chronic disease management in childhood. Again, in keeping with a developmental model, one must account for and recognize that children are acquiring cognitive skills across the life course and such skills allow them to take on increasing self-management over time. The final goal of adult self-management must be kept in mind. The shared approach has driven the service system developed in Toronto for youth in transition to adult care. The model (originally presented by Kieckhefer and Trahms[15]) depicts how the roles of health care providers, parents, and individuals change over time. The child moves from passively receiving care to active engagement and finally to management of care (as an adult). Service providers' roles change from the major care provision to consultation and finally becoming a resource. Parents' role also diminishes over time, ending as a consultant to the family member with impairment.[7]

The scarcity of adult health care providers who are knowledgeable in SB puts more responsibility on the individuals with SB and their families to prepare for adult management of SB. The adult urologist and neurosurgeon need general information about SB as well as particular information about the unique aspects of the condition in that individual. Thus, the Life Course Model has a strong emphasis on the adult goal of strong patient-directed self-management and outlines steps to prepare for such an occurrence, which is consistent with the prevailing belief of empowerment that undergirds the adult disability movement. Admittedly, this self-management pushes the limits by encouraging what might be viewed by some as an unwelcomed intrusion into medical care by patients. But this tension is welcomed by others as a reflection of changing paradigms, needed to accompany the longer life and higher aspirations of people with disabilities. The driving force behind the Life Course Model is echoed in the statement on self-determination:

Self-Determination is both person-centered and person-directed. It acknowledges the rights of people with disabilities to take charge of and responsibility for their lives. In Self-Determination, the individual, not the service system, decides where he or she will live, and with whom; what type of services he or she requires, and who will provide them; how he or she will spend his or her time, which may include the type of vocational or educational opportunities he or she wishes to engage in, and how he or she will relate to the community, which may include joining in community events, taking part in civic groups, and developing and maintaining relationships with others in the community.[6]

SUMMARY

Empowerment and self-determination have become dominant themes for adults with disabilities. Parents and their children with disabilities can see examples of how adults are doing to guide the management of their lives, including health self-management, and to motivate them for full participation in adulthood. Examples of typical childhood development serve as a guide to preparing for adult life.

The trajectory to full participation may be lower and slower, but one needs to be established. A developmental approach is needed to map trajectory to successful participation.

Self-management of health conditions is especially important when adult health care providers lack knowledge of adult patients with pediatric onset chronic conditions and disabilities.

CHALLENGES AND OPPORTUNITIES POSED BY THE LIFE COURSE MODEL

For many health care providers, the Life Course Model is a new paradigm, whereby functional adult outcomes become the goal of traditional management of body systems. Tracking and measuring progress in these domains may seem subjective. Better measures of participation need to be developed at all stages of development. Intentionally sharing condition management with parents and ultimately with the child may be a shift in approach to some health care providers.

For individuals and families, the Life Course Model forces a focus on long-term outcomes: what will happen when the child becomes an adult. Initially, families often focus on their own loss and grief. When the child is born (even earlier, if the diagnosis is known before delivery), the family faces the reality of having a child with lifelong impairment and its possible consequences. Just getting through the first few years of medical issues, such as hydrocephalus/shunting, is demanding. When the child stabilizes medically, the family can start looking forward to the more distant events, preschool and school. Providers and support persons can help inch the family toward the long view of adult life and reinforce the steps that can be taken in the present to prepare for the future. Showing a pathway to adult life through the Life Course Model can help families see that there is a step-by-step process that can be broken down into manageable steps across the life course. Families can learn that each milestone builds on a previous one and that participation in adulthood is attainable.

Although this article and issue focus on SB as a sentinel condition conducive to the Life Course Model, the model can be easily applied to all chronic conditions of childhood onset. Regardless of how the impairments are clustered in a specific condition or in an individual, the principles of preparation for adult participation through the use of a Life Course Model can be adopted and implemented by all affected families and their health care providers.

REFERENCES

1. Prabhakar H, Haywood C Jr, Molokie R. Sickle cell disease in the United States: looking back and forward at 100 years of progress in management and survival. Am J Hematol 2010;85(5):346–53.
2. Gomez-Merino E, Bach JR. Duchenne muscular dystrophy: prolongation of life by noninvasive ventilation and mechanically assisted coughing. Am J Phys Med Rehabil 2002;81(6):411–5.
3. Bowman RM, McLone DG, Grant JA, et al. Spina bifida outcome: a 25-year prospective. Pediatr Neurosurg 2001;34(3):114–20.
4. Cystic Fibrosis Foundation. Patient registry: annual data report 2008. Bethesda (MD): Cystic Fibrosis Foundation; 2008.
5. Roebroeck ME, Jahnsen R, Carona C, et al. Adult outcomes and lifespan issues for people with childhood-onset physical disability. Dev Med Child Neurol 2009; 51(8):670–8.
6. National Resource Center for Self Determination Web site. Available at: http://thechp.syr.edu/determination.pdf. Accessed June 10, 2010.
7. Gall C, Kingsworth S, Healy H. Growing up ready: a shared management approach. Phys Occup Ther Pediatr 2006;26(4):47–56.
8. Perrin EC, Gerrity SG. Development of children with a chronic illness. Pediatr Clin North Am 1984;31(1):19–31.
9. ICF Web site. Available at: http://apps.who.int/classifications/icfbrowser/. Accessed June 10, 2010.
10. Chung RJ, Burke PJ, Goodman E. Firm foundations: strength-based approaches to adolescent chronic disease. Curr Opin Pediatr 2010;22(4):389–97.
11. Jessen ED, Colver AF, Mackie PC, et al. Development and validation of a tool to measure the impact of childhood disabilities on the lives of children and their families. Child Care Health Dev 2003;29(1):21–34.
12. McConachie H, Colver AF, Forsyth RJ, et al. Participation of disabled children: how should it be characterized and measured? Disabil Rehabil 2006;28(13):1157–64.

13. Coster W, Khetani MA. Measuring participation of children with disabilities: issues and challenges. Disabil Rehabil 2008;30(8):639–48.
14. Von Korff M, Gruman J, Schaefer J, et al. Collaborative management of chronic illness. Ann Intern Med 1997;127(12):1097–102.
15. Kieckhefer GM, Trahms CM. Supporting development of children with chronic conditions: from compliance towards shared management. Pediatr Nurs 2000; 26:354–63.

The National Spina Bifida Program Transition Initiative: The People, the Plan, and the Process

Judy K. Thibadeau, RN, MN[a],*,
Ann I. Alriksson-Schmidt, PhD, MSPH[a],
T. Andrew Zabel, PhD, ABPP[b,c]

KEYWORDS

- Spina bifida • Transition • Health care • Social relationships
- Employment

Spina bifida (SB) is a multidimensional condition thought to impact different life-domains across the course of development. Children born three to four decades ago who were affected by chronic childhood conditions, such as SB and cerebral palsy, generally did not live to adulthood.[1] Survival rates for conditions such as these have increased dramatically in industrialized countries since that time[2] and are no longer considered to result in premature death by default. Nevertheless, growing up with SB or cerebral palsy poses multiple challenges that children without a chronic and complex disabling condition do not experience. Thus, the manner in which SB-related variables influence the transition of youth into adulthood has increasingly become an area of public health interest.

Preparing for life as an adult for any young person with such conditions involves a broad range of concerns, inevitable stumbling blocks, as well as opportunities for creative adaptation. Current understanding of the condition-related impact of SB

This work was supported by the National Spina Bifida Program, National Center on Birth Defects and Developmental Disabilities, Centers for Disease Control and Prevention, Atlanta, Georgia.

The authors have nothing to disclose.

[a] Division of Human Development and Disability, National Center on Birth Defects and Developmental Disabilities, Centers for Disease Control and Prevention, 1600 Clifton Road, NE MS E-88, Atlanta, GA 30333, USA

[b] Department of Neuropsychology, Philip A. Keelty Center for Spina Bifida and Related Conditions, Kennedy Krieger Institute, 1750 East Fairmount Avenue, Baltimore, MD 21231, USA

[c] Department of Psychiatry and Behavioral Science, Johns Hopkins University School of Medicine, 733 North Broadway, Baltimore, MD 21205, USA

* Corresponding author.

E-mail address: csn2@cdc.gov

upon transition processes includes several promising areas of knowledge, but also includes significant research gaps and domains that have been understudied, leaving in many instances decisions to be made based on personal expert opinions. However, research has shown that, in addition to the perhaps obvious medical complications that can occur with complex childhood conditions compared with adolescents without physical disabilities, 11- to 16-year-old adolescents with physical disabilities reported more difficulty with decision making, more difficulty making and communicating with friends, that they were less likely to have plans to attend college, and more likely to be unable to express what they would be doing at age sixteen.[3] Moreover, challenges were also reported in achieving independent living, vocational independence, and community mobility, and in participation in social activities.[3] Although the value that is placed on having a job, living independently, and having hobbies and friends is subjective and, to some degree, culture-specific, they are generally important cornerstones in people's lives.

The Centers for Disease Control and Prevention (CDC) has a long and successful history in the discovery of causative factors of SB and in the prevention of births that are affected by SB.[4] However, it was not until 2003 that a more coordinated CDC effort was initiated to include a focus on persons who are born and living with SB. The National Spina Bifida Program (NSBP) was developed as a congressionally mandated program and placed at the National Center for Birth Defects and Developmental Disabilities at CDC. The goals of this program are to: facilitate independence, enhance participation in society, increase access to effective health care, and to increase the number of persons living healthy lives with minimal associated health conditions. To achieve these goals, surveillance, intramural and extramural research, close collaboration with SB advocacy organizations such as the Spina Bifida Association (SBA), as well as other mechanisms and partnerships are used.

Many believe that to realize the desired level of independence and participation by adults with SB, intentional preparation for this achievement needs to begin at an early age.[5] However, although it is mandated that aging out of the school system be preceded by "transition" planning, this planning generally occurs when a child reaches the age of 14 to 15 years. The plan typically encompasses what he or she may be doing upon leaving high school—work, further education, or some type of training. Although the condition-related impact of SB is better understood during early periods of child development, it is considerably less well understood during adolescence and young adulthood and there is little research or guidance on how to manage the transition process. Even in well-designed research studies, there is often little linkage between findings and eventual outcomes that might be useful for guiding interventions to improve the outcomes of the adult transition process in SB. The American Academy of Pediatrics has expended much effort to describe the need for and the difficulties associated with the transfer to a health care system that is family-centered, continuous, comprehensive, coordinated, compassionate, and culturally competent for children with special health care needs as they become too old to be cared for in the pediatric system of care.[6] The term "transition" has been used to refer to this transfer of medical care effort as well. However, the issues of transition are much broader and long-standing than either of these definitions and require the interplay of medical, educational, and social systems that are often working independently and not set up to support the achievement of independence or the early and ongoing developmental work that may be necessary for a successful transition into young adulthood for persons living with chronic childhood conditions. The creation of a resource to guide the preparation for adult participation (ie, life-course transitioning) was consequently identified as a high priority area by the NSBP. The availability of a resource of this kind will help individuals with SB as well as their parents, teachers, doctors, and other professionals anticipate common SB-related developmental challenges as well as obtain information regarding known intervention or accommodation approaches.

THE PROCESS OF THE NSBP TRANSITION INITIATIVE

The concept of delineating the problems and developing a plan to be used to facilitate the life-course transition process for persons with SB, and possibly other chronic childhood conditions, was developed by NSBP professionals. The first step involved organizing a two-day Transition Summit hosted by CDC. Persons living with SB and family members of persons living with SB, as well as professionals from different disciplines with recognized expertise in SB and SB research (including developmental pediatrics, nursing, psychology, occupational therapy, and rehabilitation medicine) were invited to participate in the Summit. Professionals representing SBA and CDC also participated. The group was charged with specific tasks. Initially, the group members were asked to state the needs of persons with SB (and other chronic childhood conditions) that must be met in order that they may transition successfully from a child-oriented system of care and services to one focused on the needs of an independent and participating adult. The discussion was then directed to describe the barriers that prevent developmentally appropriate transitions throughout the life course in medical and nonmedical areas; to describe interventions or programs with demonstrated success in addressing the identified barriers to successful and timely transitions; and to describe the expected outcomes of effective transition programs or resources. Toward the end of the Transition Summit, a conversation was held to identify the next steps needed to put available and appropriate transition-related resources into the hands of persons who may need them. To frame this work, the NSBP's draft "Life-Course Model" (discussed in detail later) was presented as a way to organize the discussion about resources and interventions. The discussion regarding interventions encompassed several specific domains that included: Health Care, Access and Use; Health Promotion; Sexuality and Reproductive Concerns; Self-Advocacy or Self-Care Management; Education or Job Training; Relationships; Socialization or Social Skills; Depression and Mental Health (including during major disasters); Transportation; Mobility; Family Interventions; and Preventing Secondary Conditions. The Transition Summit discussions resulted in the articulation of a number of key principles to guide the development of interventions, as well as the identification of interventions specific to particular age groups. A summary of these key principles is presented in **Box 1.**

Following the Transition Summit, NSBP elicited a one-year commitment from each of the Summit participants who were willing and able to continue working on the transition initiative. The group in its entirety (20) consented to the one-year commitment. A timeline representing the overall progress of the work is outlined in **Fig. 1.**

The Life-Course Model for Spina Bifida

The life problems experienced by a person and the impact of those problems are unique to each individual and his or her specific situation and condition. Recommendations to buffer or solve the problems encountered would, of course, include an assessment of each person's situation, desires, and life circumstances. Nevertheless, there are certain key domains that, without consideration throughout the life course, may result in a less than satisfactory progression to independence, participation, and health. The consistent mantra throughout this work has been that to successfully prepare a young adult for a healthy life that includes participation and self-sufficiency.

Box 1
Key concepts from the transition summit

General

- Transition begins early—identify developmental issues at birth and across the life course.
- Monitor developmental progress systematically in different stages or aspects of life.
- Individualize transition interventions as appropriate and based on developmental assessment.

Adolescents

- Begin planning for transition before child becomes an adolescent.
- Education and guidance for adolescents is essential. Information should be provided often and until the adolescent models behavior that is reflective of the education.
- At times, male or female differences and concerns may need to be addressed in same-gender groups.
- Mentor teens with SB by adults with SB.
- Create opportunities for participation in team sports and group activities.
- Create and use peer groups.

Young Adults

- Empower young adults to be self-advocates
- Link young adults to offices of disability at post-secondary schools
- Promote volunteerism and building and sustaining relationships

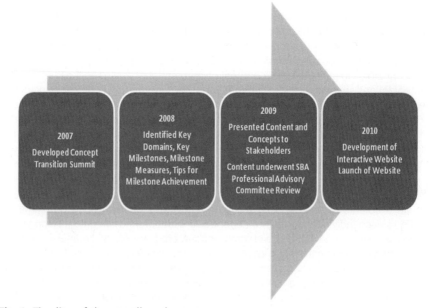

Fig. 1. Timeline of the overall work progress.

Intentional preparation needs to begin at an early age. Therefore, the Life-Course Model was laid out developmentally, beginning with the preschool years and continuing through school-age, adolescence, and young adulthood. It is acknowledged that an individual's development does not end at young adulthood. However, it became necessary to put parameters on the work because it quickly became extensive, and there were concerns that it would become overwhelming and unwieldy for the work groups and for the final user.

The Life-Course Model was designed to address three broad functional domains: Health and Condition Self Management; Social and Personal Relationships; and Education or Income Support (**Fig. 2**).

The first of these broad functional dimensions, Health and Condition Self Management, included discrete functional domains related to mobility, skin integrity, sexuality, obesity prevention, bowel or bladder management, and condition self-management. The second broad functional domain area was Social and Personal Relationships, which included content specific to discrete functional domains including the personal development of the individual with SB, as well as his or her relationship with parents, siblings, friends, and romantic or intimate partners. The third and final broad functional domain was Education or Income Support, which included a focus upon discrete areas such as cognitive development, mastery of different academic content, functional academics, prevocational skill development, and the development of responsibility-taking behaviors. Discrete functional domains were identified within each of these broad functional areas, and these discrete areas were further subdivided by age to examine smaller transitional steps occurring within each discrete functional domain during the preschool, school-age, adolescent, and young adult time periods. Segmentation of discrete functional domains according to broad age ranges permitted a greater appreciation of the transition processes occurring across the development of youth with SB. For instance, examining the development of condition self-management skills according to the noted age ranges helped elucidate a series of transitional steps that would be useful for focusing research and intervention efforts.

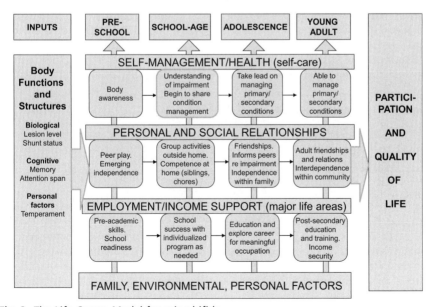

Fig. 2. The Life-Course Model for spina bifida.

Examples include: beginning awareness of SB during preschool, engagement in health promotion and illness prevention during the school-age years, gradual reduction in need for external self care supervision and prompting during adolescence, and eventual independence in self-management and self-care competencies during young adulthood. In the end, examining transition of youth with SB via both the age dimension and the functional dimension proved useful for identifying distinct and parallel developmental processes thought to underlie the gradual transition of youth with SB into the roles and responsibilities of adulthood.

The Life-Course Model also incorporates unique factors that each person with SB or other chronic condition brings to the table. These factors were delineated as biologic factors, personal factors, and cognitive skills. Common to these factors is that they are not very, if at all, modifiable. Other factors certainly have the potential to moderate outcomes, such as family, environment, and culture. These factors may or may not be modifiable, but they are likely to impact how the other factors interact. Although the vital role of these potential moderating factors was acknowledged in the model, they were not explored or developed in any detail.

The Life-Course Model proved helpful in organizing the different topics that the working groups (discussed in more detail later) identified as the issues most relevant to facilitate the timely and successful path through the developmental stages and it has continued to be useful to summarize the completed work. It cannot, and is not intended to be, an all encompassing transition model.

There are clear similarities between the International Classification of Functioning Disability and Health (ICF)[7] and the Life-Course Model although the terminology and the purpose differ. Whereas the ICF is a detailed classification system for the description of health and health-related states, the Life-Course Model was designed to specifically target the process and actions needed for multiple life stages and life-course transition for persons with SB. Nevertheless, what are referred to as "inputs" in the Life-Course Model are comparable to, for example, "body functions and structure" and "personal factors" in the ICF. Both models also acknowledge the importance of environmental factors as well as participation in life and society. With participation and quality of life as the long-term goals, the work groups populated the different cells in the Life-Course Model by domain and age group, with concepts that were considered to represent key developmental milestones, measures and indicators of milestone achievement, tips to accomplish the key milestone, and associated references.

TRANSITION WORKING GROUPS

After the Transition Summit and as a result of the themes that emerged during the Summit that were important to the successful transition of persons affected by SB, five working groups were created (**Fig. 3**).

Each group consisted of four to five people and a volunteer leader. The leader, in conjunction with professionals from CDC, organized the work and facilitated the progress. The groups worked via conference calls from November, 2007, until June, 2008, reviewing the literature and determining their approach to develop a Life-Course Model of transition. In addition, the group leaders held a separate conference call monthly to discuss progress and differences in approach. During this time the groups recommended the final product be developed into an interactive Web site that could be used by parents of children born with SB, persons with SB, and professionals working with persons affected by SB. Although the focus was clearly on SB, many in the working groups recognized the overlap of this work with the process of transition

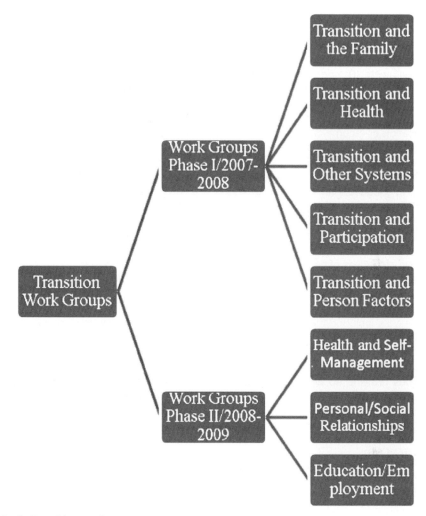

Fig. 3. Transition work groups.

for children with other chronic childhood conditions. Therefore, the literature reviews that were undertaken were not limited to SB. The groups had a second face-to-face meeting in Tucson, Arizona, at the annual national SBA meeting at which time they shared the status of the work on their topics. After the meeting, the five groups were restructured into three groups that would encompass the aspects included in the initial domains: Health or Condition Self Management; Social and Personal Relationships; and Education or Income Support (see **Fig. 3**). These groups worked from November, 2008, until June, 2009, at which time, during the SBA Annual Meeting, the three domains were highlighted in specific presentations to receive feedback from clinicians, persons with SB, and their families regarding the relevance and the content of the model and the domains. The sessions were well received; comments were recorded and incorporated into a final version of the Life-Course Model. The work was also vetted with attendants at the First World Congress on Spina Bifida in Orlando, Florida, in March of 2009.

The final version of the document underwent a review by a subcommittee of the SBA Professional Advisory Committee. Comments received were considered and incorporated as appropriate and the Spina Bifida Life-Course Model was finalized. This content is being incorporated by SBA into a Web-version for access by clinicians, persons with SB, and their families, and will be available via the SBA Web site late in 2010. A key recommendation of the working groups is that the information not be presented so as to be too voluminous at one time. Therefore, users may access the content by domain (Health or Self Management, Personal or Social Relationships, Education or Income Support) or by age (preschool, school-age, adolescent, young adult), and navigate through the site viewing as much or as little content as desired. Incorporated into the Web application is the opportunity for the reader to answer questions regarding the developmental progress of a person in the different domains so as to gauge roughly the progress made toward the achievement of a specific developmental milestone. It should be noted, however, that the Web site is organized to efficiently summarize information that may be applicable to a person. It is not a standardized self-assessment and should not be regarded as such. It is intended to be complementary to, and not replace, the work and advice of health care professionals in the lives of persons affected by SB. Individuals who access the Web site will have the opportunity to share personal success stories and helpful tips and interventions that may be used to assist others to make progress toward achieving the particular milestones. The site will be reviewed on at least an annual basis for the verification of the links included as well as to provide an opportunity for information review and update.

This article outlines and summarizes the rationale and the work process that was undertaken to address the issues of transitioning throughout the life course for persons growing up with SB. Although this work focused specifically on transition for children and adolescents with SB, there is substantial overlap with other chronic childhood complex conditions.

REFERENCES

1. Binks JA, Barden WS, Burke TA, et al. What do we really know about the transition to adult-centered health care? A focus on cerebral palsy and spina bifida. Arch Phys Med Rehabil 2007;88:1064–73.
2. White P. Essential components of programs for transition to adulthood. American experience. Rev Rhum Engl Ed 1997;64(Suppl 10):198S–9S.
3. Stevens SE, Steele CA, Jutai JW, et al. Adolescents with physical disabilities: some psychosocial aspects of health. J Adolesc Health 1996;19(2):157–64.
4. Centers for Disease Control. Recommendations for the use of folic acid to reduce the number of cases of spina bifida and other neural tube defects. MMWR Recomm Rep 1992;41(RR-14):1–7.
5. Peterson PM, Rauen KK, Brown J, et al. Spina bifida: the transition into adulthood begins in infancy. Rehabil Nurs 1994;19(4):229–38.
6. American Academy of Pediatrics; American Academy of Family Physicians; American College of Physicians-American Society of Internal Medicine. A consensus statement on health care transitions for young adults with special health care needs. Pediatrics 2002;110:1304–6.
7. World Health Organization. International classification of functioning, disability and health. Geneva (Switzerland): World Health Organization; 2001.

The Life Course Model Web Site: An Online Transition-Focused Resource for the Spina Bifida Community

T. Andrew Zabel, PhD, ABPP[a,b,*], Ronna Linroth, PhD, OT[c], Andrea D. Fairman, MOT, OTR/L, CPRP[d,e]

KEYWORDS

• Spina bifida • Transition • Adulthood • Development

Spina bifida (SB) is a multi-dimensional disorder thought to impact different life domains across the course of development. The manner in which SB-related variables influence the transition of youth into adulthood has increasingly become an area of public health interest, particularly given medical advances that have made survival into adulthood the general rule rather than the exception.[1] Current understanding of the disease-related impact of SB upon these transition processes includes several promising areas of knowledge, but also includes significant research gaps and domains that have been understudied (see the article by Kathleen Sawin elsewhere in this issue for further exploration of this topic). The disease-related impact of SB is best understood in domains such as education,[2,3] and is far less understood in

---

[a] Department of Neuropsychology, Philip A. Keelty Center for Spina Bifida and Related Conditions, Kennedy Krieger Institute, 801 North Broadway, Baltimore, MD 21205, USA
[b] Department of Psychiatry and Behavioral Science, Johns Hopkins University School of Medicine, 733 North Broadway, Baltimore, MD 21205, USA
[c] Adult Outpatient Services, Gillette Lifetime Specialty Healthcare, 435 Phalen Boulevard, St Paul, MN 55130, USA
[d] Adult Spina Bifida Clinic, Department of Physical Medicine and Rehabilitation, University of Pittsburgh Medical Center (UPMC), Kaufmann Medical Building, Suite 202, 3471 5th Avenue, Pittsburgh, PA 15213, USA
[e] Department of Rehabilitation Science and Technology, University of Pittsburgh, School of Health and Rehabilitation Sciences, Forbes Tower, Suite 5044, 3600 Forbes Avenue, Pittsburgh, PA 15260, USA
* Corresponding author. Department of Psychiatry and Behavioral Science, Johns Hopkins University School of Medicine, Baltimore, MD.
E-mail address: zabela@kennedykrieger.org

Pediatr Clin N Am 57 (2010) 911–917
doi:10.1016/j.pcl.2010.07.011
0031-3955/10/$ – see front matter © 2010 Elsevier Inc. All rights reserved.

domains such as employment and independent living in adulthood. Similarly, disease-related impact of SB is better understood during early periods of child development,[4] and is considerably less well understood during adolescence and young adulthood. Moreover, even in well designed studies, there is often little linkage between research findings and eventual outcomes that might be useful for guiding interventions to improve the outcomes of the adult transition process in SB.

This combination of islands of fruitful transition-related research mixed with significant research gaps/understudied areas has increased the difficulty associated with developing integrated lifespan resources for individuals with SB. The Life Course Model Web site project was initiated in 2007 by the Centers for Disease Control and Prevention and the Spina Bifida Association to accumulate SB-related transition-related information and organize it into a useful and accessible resource (see the article by Thibadeau and colleagues elsewhere in this issue for further exploration of this topic). Specifically, this effort was intended to help individuals with SB as well as their parents, teachers, doctors, and other professionals anticipate common SB-related developmental challenges and to obtain information regarding known intervention and accommodation approaches. The overall design is intended to facilitate an individualized exploration of information specific to the different functional transitions presented to youth with SB as they develop, and then to provided associated intervention tips and resources from the available research and the large body of experience of parents and clinicians in the field.

STRUCTURE OF THE LIFE COURSE MODEL WEB SITE

The specialized transition-related information included in the Life Course Model Web site is organized around the Life Course Model described by Mark E. Swanson in this issue. This model includes four general age ranges; preschool, school-age, adolescence, and young adulthood. Each of these age ranges was noted to contain important transitions in multiple functional life domains. For instance, important academic transitions are experienced by most individuals with SB in each of the noted age ranges, including the beginning of formal schooling, the transition of the individual into the increased academic expectations of third and fourth grade, the transition of the individual into middle school/high school, and the process involved in making plans following high school. Other transition processes can be traced along this time dimension, such as the series of transitions that occur within the parent/child relationship (eg, the development of parent/child attachment in childhood, a gradual shift of responsibilities from parent to child in adolescence, and the eventual development of parent/child interdependence in young adulthood).

In addition to the age clusters described, the logic model that provides the underlying structure to the Life Course Model Web site also includes several broad functional domains that represent another dimension of the model. The first of these broad functional dimensions, self-management/health, includes discrete functional domains related to mobility, skin integrity, sexuality, obesity prevention, bowel/bladder management, and condition self-management. The second broad functional domain area is personal and social relationships; this area includes content specific to discrete functional domains, including the personal development of the individual with SB, as well as his or her relationship with parents, siblings, friends, and romantic/intimate partners. The third and final broad functional domain of the Life Course Model Web site is employment and income support; this area includes a focus upon discrete areas such as cognitive development, mastery of different academic content, functional academics, prevocational skill development, and the development of responsibility-taking behaviors. Discrete functional domains are identified within each of these broad functional areas, and these discrete areas are further subdivided by age to examine smaller transitional steps occurring within each discrete functional domain during the preschool, school-age, adolescent, and young adult time periods.

The Life Course Model Web site allows exploration of the noted SB-related transition information according to both age dimension and the functional dimension, thereby demonstrating the distinct and parallel developmental processes thought to underlie the gradual transition of youth with SB into the roles and responsibilities of adulthood. Specifically, the Web site format allows an exploration of a distinct functional domain (eg, relationship with siblings) sequentially by age (ie, longitudinally), allowing one to see the conceptual manner in which this distinct functional domain develops across the lifespan (eg, managing early sibling conflicts during the school-aged years may facilitate the development of mutual sibling support during young adulthood). The flexibility of the Web-based format also allows for exploration of the functional domain by individual age ranges (ie, cross-sectional), allowing one to see the manner in which distinct functional domain elements might overlap, develop in tandem, or mutually facilitate growth at different periods of time (eg, maximizing mobility during preschool may help prevent obesity during preschool).

The Life Course Model Web site is intended to allow navigation of the transition content in a number of different ways based upon the user's individual concerns, learning styles, or interests. To organize content areas, specific indicators of milestone achievement are included by age and functional domain. These indicators of developmental progress allow the user to quickly assess the developmental gains of his or her child with SB within the context of the transition model. For instance, a parent of a preschooler can quickly access indicators of success transitional achievement during the preschool years, and use this information to gauge a child's progress or needs. In turn, the same parent of a preschooler with SB can review indicators of discrete functional development during childhood and adolescence, perhaps in anticipation of upcoming transitional challenges and developmental steps. To facilitate access to these indicators of milestone achievement, the indicators of milestone achievement are worded in question format, which facilitates the possibility of an online developmental survey that can help direct parents, teachers, clinicians, and others to indicators and content that may be of particular interest based upon their survey responses.

In addition to the milestones and indicators described previously, the Life Course Model Web site presents various practical tips, intervention strategies, and assessment techniques that are associated with the indicators/milestones in the transition process. There are currently few (if any) evidenced-based practices that have been developed for addressing the academic, personal/social, or health care and self-management needs of youth with SB. As such, most tips and intervention strategies are generated out of either promising practices or reports of effectiveness based upon parent or clinician anecdotal report. The Web-based platform allows all of these tips and intervention strategies to be available for review at any point at which a parent, clinician, or person with SB encounters a discrete functional content area for which he or she wants intervention advice. In this respect, the tips and interventions are nested within the broader transition related content, and the interested user can access this information via a simple mouse click. Furthermore, link-out options permit direct electronic routing of the user to additional Internet-based resources such as scientific abstracts, source documents, additional explanations of concepts, or additional resources in areas of interest or concern.

In short, the Web site model allows the user to navigate horizontally among the indicators of milestone achievement in different functional domain areas and during various periods of development, but also allows the user to drill down into the Web site for helpful tips and strategies for addressing indicator-related areas of concern. The following examples are presented to illustrate this drill down process. These examples were selected to illustrate the age range included in the Life Course Model Web site (preschool, school age, adolescence, young adulthood), provide examples of the functional domains, and demonstrate the organization of the content included.

EXAMPLE OF WEB SITE USE: PRESCHOOL, SOCIAL DEVELOPMENT

The distal outcomes of SB in young adulthood are increasingly believed to be shaped in part by earlier developmental transition processes, and the transition content of the Life Course Model Web site extends down to the preschool years to reflect this early influence. The preschool years are a particularly salient period in which play and friendship skills develop, and preschoolers with SB often have the added barrier of physical/mobility-related issues that disrupt aspects of preschool peer interactions.

A parent, teacher, or day care provider could find considerable information about the social development of preschoolers with SB on the Life Course Model Web site, including several indicators that could help determine if a youngster is meeting key social milestones such as the transition from parallel to interactive play. The transition to interactive play is a key component to social competence and acceptance, and can be an area of difficulty for preschoolers with SB. To help assess this, the Web site user is cued to answer several preschool-related questions, such as

Does your child appear comfortable in small play groups?
Does your child share some toys with peers?
Does your child seem to understand the feelings of other children?

Answering yes to these questions provides age-related feedback and assurance regarding milestone achievement, and answering no highlights a potential area for additional assessment or intervention.

If concerned about this social milestone, a parent or educational provider could easily drill down in the Web site content at this point and access intervention-related information to help create opportunities for further social interaction. For instance, intervention strategies might include providing the child with SB access to a play group, and providing other parents or teachers with information about SB to assure them that safe interactive play with preschoolers with SB is both possible and necessary. Similarly, tips and interventions at this level include guidance to help potential peers understand and demystify SB by bringing SB-related items to the playgroup (eg, wheelchairs), talking about the items with children in the play group, and letting the other preschoolers ride in them. Both of these intervention approaches are designed to help provide the preschooler with SB access to social settings by helping parents, teachers, and other children better understand the condition. In this instance, the interventions are targeted toward helping to reduce the fear or uncertainty experienced by others regarding SB, and allow them to comfortably interact with children with SB. Assuring other parents and other children that SB is nothing to be afraid of will then set the stage for more opportunities for interactive play.

EXAMPLE OF WEB SITE USE: SCHOOL AGE, OBESITY PREVENTION

Many of the health outcomes of SB evolve over time, with early medical status, procedures, and preventative care occurring during childhood thought to shape the health outcomes in youth adulthood. The Life Course Model Web site includes many indicators of health-related milestone achievement that can help families and medical teams gauge the extent to which a child with SB is developing in a way that will support positive health outcomes in the future. One particularly salient area of health-related concern for youth with SB during childhood is obesity prevention, as intervention efforts to prevent obesity can help prevent many other conditions (pressure sores) with downsteam implications for health status in young adulthood. Within the Life Course Model Web site, a primary developmental milestone for children with SB involves maintaining appropriate weight for height and age. The Life Course Model Web site provides information and links to help professionals assess this developmental milestone and monitor weight and body mass index. Moreover, the Life Course Model site provides multiple questions to help the provider, parent, or nurse determine if the child is showing other indicators of healthy weight management for age.

For instance, involvement in physical activity is an important secondary indicator of obesity prevention efforts, and the preparation site queries the parent or health care provider on issues such as exercise (Does your child participate in adapted physical education at school?) and sports involvement (Is your child a member of a community adapted sports team?). If the respondent answers no to the first of these questions, he or she can drill down in the Web site to find multiple resources regarding adapted physical education, including resources for adapted physical education teachers, guidance regarding the use of paraeducators for physical education class, and suggestions for assessing the child's present level of performance and developing appropriate child-specific adaptive physical education (APE) goals.

Similarly, if the parent, teacher, or health professional answered no to questions about the child's involvement with an adapted sports team, he or she would have the option of drilling down in the Web site to additional resources and suggestions regarding this type of activity. These resources include a rationale for athletic involvement (eg, self-confidence, self-reliance, independence, problem-solving abilities, and leadership skills), sports readiness assessment sheets for various wheelchair sports, links for searching (by state) for adapted sports programs and camps, and links to fan sites for paraathletes. In this manner, indicators of obesity prevention are brought to the attention of parents, educators, and medical professionals, and these individuals can help steer children with SB into adapted physical education or adapted sports programs.

EXAMPLE OF WEB SITE USE: ADOLESCENCE, CONDITION MANAGEMENT/SELF-CARE

In individuals with SB, condition self-management involves the individual's knowledge base concerning SB and his or her ability to engage in activities related to personal safety, medication management, and complication prevention. This is an important area of transition concentration, as responsibility for condition management progressively shifts from the parent to the individual with SB over time. Adolescence is a particularly salient period of time in this transition, as condition management is thought to become the primary responsibility of the adolescent with SB, and the parent progressively moves into a supportive (rather than primary) role.

The adolescent transition milestones of the Life Course Model Web site reflect this shift (eg, the adolescent is independent in self care or care management with or without supervision and prompting), and the questions presented to the user provide further indication as to whether this transition is occurring. For instance, indicator questions query whether the adolescent can initiate making a medical appointment, asks basic questions of health care providers, reports pain episodes including headaches, monitors status of supplies and medications before they run out, and takes medicines without prompting or cues.

If the answer to any of these questions is no, the user of the Web site further delves into the available resources, tips, and interventions linked to each of the indicator questions described previously. For example, links to products designed to help improve management of medication and medical appointments are provided, including links to resources such as equipment order flow sheets and talking with your doctor video clips. If an adolescent with SB is struggling to assume more responsibility for medication and other self-care responsibilities, the Life Course Model Web site provides links to multiple transition assessment tools, guides to SB, and health care transition workbooks.

EXAMPLE OF WEB SITE USE: YOUNG ADULTHOOD, ACTIVITIES OF DAILY LIVING

One of the most challenging of transitions faced by individuals with SB is the move from a supported home environment into a living setting with far fewer prompts, cues, or reminders to complete essential aspects of independent living. Transitioning in this manner requires independent initiation, completion of activities of daily living, and taking responsibility for household matters. In addition to condition management and medically related self-care, movement into a less restrictive/supportive setting presents the challenge of organizing the routine aspects of daily life. The Life Course Model Web site can be a useful resource for anticipating the challenges the young adult with SB will face when transitioning out of the family home setting, or assessing his or her progress once he or she has taken on more responsibility for the activities of daily living.

To help assess how well the young adult with SB is taking responsibility for independent living skills, the Life Course Model Web site provides several cueing questions. These questions focus upon topics such as making and keeping appointments, preparing meals, doing housework, and managing finances. In the event that the Web site user indicates that any or all of these topics are areas of concern, he or she can identify specific assessment methods that can further delineate specific areas of independent living strengths and weaknesses. Moreover, there are multiple tips and intervention strategies listed that are frequently found useful by individuals with SB when taking on more responsibilities, including guidance for using technologies such as timers and alarms, pill box organizers, smartphones, on-line reminder services, voice recorders, and talking key chains. Additionally, recommendations of specific accommodative devices are provided, including different reminder systems engineered for individuals with cognitive disabilities.

SUMMARY

The transition of youth with SB into adulthood is an exciting opportunity to branch out, explore and participate in community, and reach higher levels of independence. The Life Course Model Web site is a resource designed to help in this process, both by confirming the progress made by individuals with SB as well as highlighting possible areas of needed accommodation or intervention. Effective Web-based presentation of this type of content is typically dynamic in nature, and is developed via multiple iterations based upon feedback regarding usability and the intuitive nature of the interface. The Web site developed out of the Life Course Model content will require periodic reworking of both format and content to deliver the most up-to-date transition-related information to parents, clinicians, teachers, and individuals with SB. It is the hope of the multidisciplinary team of individuals behind the Life Course Model Web site that the content, format, and usability features of the site will provide a new level of accessibility to knowledge, resources, and guidance related to youth with SB, and that this information will help reduce the disease-related impact of SB upon youth as they move into the roles and responsibilities of adulthood.

ACKNOWLEDGMENTS

The authors wish to thank all members of the work groups who contributed to the development of the Web site and thus to this article.

REFERENCES

1. Bowman RM, McLone DG, Grant JA, et al. Spina bifida outcome: a 25-year prospective. Pediatr Neurosurg 2001;34(3):114–20.
2. Fletcher JM, Barnes M, Dennis M. Language development in children with spina bifida. Semin Pediatr Neurol 2002;9(3):201–8.
3. Yeates KO, Loss N, Colvin AN, et al. Do children with myelomeningocele and hydrocephalus display nonverbal learning disabilities? An empirical approach to classification. J Int Neuropsychol Soc 2003;9(4):653–62.
4. Lomax-Bream LE, Barnes M, Copeland K, et al. The impact of spina bifida on development across the first 3 years. Dev Neuropsychol 2007;31(1):1–20.

A Family Perspective: How this Product can Inform and Empower Families of Youth with Spina Bifida

Grayson N. Holmbeck, PhD[a],*,
Ann I. Alriksson-Schmidt, PhD, MSPH[b],
Melissa H. Bellin, PhD, MSW, LCSW[c], Cecily Betz, PhD, RN[d],
Katie A. Devine, PhD[a]

KEYWORDS

• Spina bifida • Youth • Family perspective

Spina bifida (SB) is a common congenital birth defect that has a significant multisystemic effect on the physical, neurocognitive, psychological, and social functioning of affected individuals. It is also well known that the clinical symptoms of SB place considerable physical, psychological, and social demands on the family members involved.[1–4] Despite the pervasive effect that this condition has on family members

Completion of this manuscript was supported in part by funding from the National Spina Bifida Program at the Centers for Disease Control and research grants from the National Institute of Child Health and Human Development (RO1 HD048629) and the March of Dimes Birth Defects Foundation (12-FY01-0098). All authors after the first are listed in alphabetical order by last name; their contributions were similar. All correspondence should be sent to: Grayson N. Holmbeck, Loyola University Chicago, Department of Psychology, 1032 W. Sheridan Road, Chicago, IL 60660 (phone: 773-508-2967; fax: 773-508-8713) (gholmbe@luc.edu).
The findings and conclusions in this article are those of the authors and do not necessarily represent the official position of the Centers for Disease Control and Prevention.
[a] Loyola University Chicago, Department of Psychology, 1032 West Sheridan Road, Chicago, IL 60660, USA
[b] National Center on Birth Defects and Developmental Disability, Division of Human Development and Disability, Centers for Disease Control and Prevention, Clifton Road, NE MS E-88, Atlanta, GA 30333, USA
[c] University of Maryland School of Social Work, 525 West Redwood Street, Baltimore, MD 21201, USA
[d] Keck School of Medicine, Department of Pediatrics, USC Center for Excellence in Developmental Disabilities, Childrens Hospital Los Angeles, 4650 Sunset Boulevard, Mail Stop #53, University of Southern California, Los Angeles, CA 90027, USA
* Corresponding author.
E-mail address: gholmbe@luc.edu

Pediatr Clin N Am 57 (2010) 919–934
doi:10.1016/j.pcl.2010.07.012
0031-3955/10/$ – see front matter © 2010 Elsevier Inc. All rights reserved.

and affected individuals, there are few family-based interventions for this at-risk population. A recent review of the literature on family interventions failed to identify any evidence-based interventions that focused on improving the psychosocial functioning of families of youth with SB.[5] Thus, the Web-based product that is the focus of this special issue is a welcome offering for families who currently lack such a resource.

Although Web-based products for families of youth with SB have not been available until now, there are family-oriented products for populations other than SB, including chronic pain, traumatic brain injury, cancer, and encopresis.[6] Research that examines the usefulness of such sites has revealed that parents and affected youth find these Web resources to be useful as they work on personal goals[7] and that their knowledge of their condition increases with increased use.[8,9] However, in some cases use has been lower than expected, perhaps because recruitment for the studies was timed inappropriately (ie, too close to diagnosis) or because the modules were too time intensive. Family use is higher if hands-on training is provided.[10]

This article focuses on how this new Web site, to be housed at the Spina Bifida Association of America (SBA) and based on the Life Course Model discussed throughout this issue, can help family members build on the strengths of individuals with SB and address areas of difficulty. Moreover, and consistent with the developmental orientation of the Life Course Model, we adopt a developmental perspective in this paper. That is, we maintain that the Life Course Model Web site is useful at all stages of development, with the information provided for families at one stage of development building on the information provided for those at earlier stages of development.

First, a brief overview is provided of relevant theories that supported the development of the Life Course Model, on which the Web site is based. Next, the literature on the adjustment of families of individuals with SB is reviewed as well as the literature on the psychosocial adjustment of affected youth. Specifically, an overview is provided of areas of difficulty for which families are most likely to seek help when using this product. We also expect that families will use the product to build on areas of existing strength. How families may benefit from engagement with the 3 content areas covered by this Web site is also discussed, namely: (1) child health and the transfer of medical management from parent to child (health/self-management), (2) the development of social relationships (social relationships), and (3) the achievement of milestones during emerging adulthood, including achievements in the areas of education and employment (education, employment, and income support).

INCORPORATION OF FAMILY-CENTERED CARE AND THE CHRONIC CARE PRINCIPLES INTO THE LIFE COURSE MODEL

The article by Swanson in this issue provides details on the conceptual thinking that incorporated principles of normal child development and the international classification of functioning, health and disability (ICF) into a framework, termed the Life Course Model. Concisely, the Life Course Model assumes: (1) for optimal development in different domains, children need to attain a sequence of milestones, which are common to all children; (2) the ICF contributes the functional domains of importance and the principle that function is an outcome of the interaction between underlying impairment (eg, cognitive deficit, leg weakness) and the surrounding environment (family, school, community).

The Life Course Model is also anchored in 2 interlocking models of health care delivery, family-centered care (FCC) and the chronic care model (CCM), both of which underscore the central importance of partnering with families to enhance medical and psychosocial outcomes for children with special health care needs, including those with SB. FCC has deep roots in the pediatric literature, particularly in research and clinical care for children with special health care needs and their families. The key elements of FCC include (1) encouraging parental involvement in decision-making; (2) fostering empowerment and self-management capacity in families; (3) attending to the needs of all members of the family unit; and (4) providing culturally respectful services.[11–13] FCC also emphasizes tailoring services to each family's identified strengths, priorities, and needs.[14,15]

This Life Course Model is consistent with the fundamental principles of FCC through its emphasis on equipping key stakeholders (including individuals with SB and their parents) with scientific data, assessment tools, and community resource information in 3 content domains: health/self-management, social relationships, and education/income support. The complementary sources of information presented on the Life Course Model Web site ideally maximize parents' capacity for informed decisions about their child's health care and position them to advocate for their child's and family's needs across the lifespan.

Establishment of the Life Course Model and construction of the Web site were similarly guided by aspects of the CCM, which suggests that productive interactions in health settings develop from "informed, activated patients and prepared, proactive practice teams."[16(p3)] Development of the CCM was sparked by increased recognition of the shortcomings of the health system in attending to psychosocial demands associated with chronic health conditions, namely the physical, social, and psychological stressors experienced by both the affected individual and surrounding family.[17] To address this apparent gap in clinical care, the CCM provides evidence-based guidelines for improving health services at multiple levels of the health system (community, organization, practice, and patient levels). Specifically, the model purports that ideal patient-provider interactions, reduced health care costs, enhanced patient satisfaction, and optimal health outcomes result from proper health care organization and delivery system design, systematic use of clinical information systems, health care provider decision support, patient and caregiver self-management support, and community linkages and resources.[18,19] Another aspect of CCM is the shared management model, in which professionals and families intentionally shift care responsibility across the life course, with the individual assuming full responsibility in adulthood.[20]

The Life Course Model Web site addresses multiple dimensions of the CCM, namely (1) provider decision support, (2) patient and caregiver self-management support, and (3) community linkages and resources. Health care providers may access the Web site to learn teaching tips as they strive to partner with individuals with SB and their families on topics of interest. Content on health/self-management, social relationships, and education/income support is presented from a lifespan perspective, which likely addresses immediate as well as long-term concerns identified by parents and individuals with SB. In the following sections, the extant literature on the adjustment of family members who have a child with SB and the psychosocial adjustment of youth with SB is reviewed, highlighting areas of difficulty that are addressed by the Life Course Model Web site. Next, how families may benefit from the Web site is outlined, including how this novel resource might maximize individual and family self-management.

REVIEW OF PAST RESEARCH ON FAMILY FUNCTIONING IN SB

Family relationships are particularly salient and influential social relationships for youth with SB, given that children with SB tend to be more socially isolated from their peers than are typically developing children.[2] Further, we are interested in family relationships because SB affects not only the child but also the parents and other family members. Given the pervasive effect of this condition, we were also interested in discussing the level of psychosocial adjustment in such individuals across multiple adjustment domains (eg, internalizing symptoms, externalizing symptoms, self-concept).

Family Functioning

Holmbeck and colleagues[5] published a review of research that examined the effect of SB on family functioning.[1,3,4,21] In general, the findings of past work support a disruption-resilience view of family functioning.[22] That is, SB seems to disrupt some aspects of family and parent functioning for many families, but such families also tend to show considerable resilience across other adjustment domains. A significant number of families in which there are children who have SB report difficulties in maintaining clear roles and responsibilities in the family system (23% in the clinically problematic range[21]). With respect to risk factors, Holmbeck and colleagues[23] found that families of youth with SB who were also from lower socioeconomic status (SES) backgrounds were particularly at risk for lower levels of family cohesion, supporting a cumulative risk view of such families (ie, SB status and lower SES have additive effects on family functioning). Given this situation, it is particularly important to market this Web site to families from low-income backgrounds and to address issues related to the availability of computer resources in this subpopulation.

Families of youth with SB do not seem to change with the development of their offspring in the same manner as is found with typically developing youth. For example, with respect to family conflicts, Coakley and colleagues[24] found that, unlike their typically developing peers, families of youth with SB did not show normative increases in family conflict as a function of pubertal development. These investigators speculated that families of youth with SB may be less responsive to developmental change. In support of this attenuated response to development hypothesis, Jandasek and colleagues[25] conducted longitudinal growth analyses in the age period of 9 to 15 years and found that family conflict intensity increased during this early adolescent age range in families of typically developing youth but not in families of children with SB. Further, parents of youth with SB are less likely to discuss issues of sexuality with their offspring than are parents of typically developing youth.[26] Therefore, this Web site aims to serve as a resource to help parents be more responsive to maturational changes in their child with SB.

Adjustment of Parents and Parenting Behaviors

Despite the low levels of family dysfunction at the family systems level, it seems that a sizable minority of parents of children with SB exhibit clinical levels of global psychological distress (eg, anxiety, depressive symptoms, somatic complaints[27,28]). Although most studies that report on parental functioning have focused on maternal functioning, one study of fathers of children with SB indicated that fathers exhibited higher levels of global distress compared with fathers from comparison families.[27] In a recent meta-analysis of 15 studies, Vermaes and colleagues[29] found medium to large effect sizes for the effect of SB on mother and father's psychological adjustment, with larger effects sizes for mothers ($d = .73$) than for fathers ($d = .54$).

Across several studies, parents of children with SB tend to experience more stress in their roles as parents than do comparison parents.[27,30,31] Typically, such parents feel less satisfied and competent as parents, feel more isolated, are less adaptable to change, and hold less optimistic views about the future than comparison parents.[27,32–34] Parents who are single, socially isolated, older, or from an ethnic minority or a low SES background are particularly at risk for such outcomes.[23,35–38]

With respect to parenting behaviors, it has been found that increases in parental responsiveness are associated with increases in adaptive coping strategies in youth with SB (eg, problem-focused coping[39]). However, parents of children with SB tend to exhibit higher levels of intrusiveness, psychological control, and authoritarian parenting (ie, parenting that undermines the autonomy development of their offspring[31,34,40–42]) and these behaviors tend to be linked with less desirable child outcomes. Specifically, higher levels of intrusiveness (sometimes referred to as over-protectiveness) tend to be associated with lower levels of decision-making autonomy, which are in turn related to higher levels of psychosocial difficulties.[34,40] Thus, parents may find this product useful in learning how to avoid certain forms of parenting that may not be beneficial to their child, which seem to be more common in families of children with SB.

Adjustment of Siblings

Few studies have examined the functioning of siblings of children with SB. Findings have been contradictory: an early study using teacher reporting found a 4-fold greater likelihood of adjustment problems for siblings relative to a comparison sample,[43] whereas a later study of siblings of youth with SB reported no differences in self-concept compared with siblings of typically developing youth.[44] Qualitative research has identified both positive and negative outcomes related to having a sibling with SB. For example, siblings report significant levels of concern for the health of their sibling with SB, emotional upset in relation to their sibling's experience with discrimination, teasing, and bullying, and sadness related to the lack of opportunities to engage in physical activities with their sibling with SB.[45,46] Siblings have also identified some positive effects, such as increased empathy for their sibling and a greater appreciation for their own physical abilities.[45,46]

The behavioral and psychological functioning of siblings has been found to be significantly associated with SES, family cohesion, perceptions of social support, and their knowledge of and attitudes toward the illness.[47–49] For siblings of children with SB, more positive attitudes toward SB, greater family satisfaction, lower levels of sibling conflict, and increased social support from classmates significantly predicted higher levels of self-concept and prosocial behavior, and lower rates of behavior problems.[50] In this study by Bellin and colleagues,[50] family satisfaction was the only significant predictor across all 3 sibling adjustment outcome measures, suggesting that family variables may be particularly salient for sibling adjustment. Therefore, parents of youth with SB may also use this Web site tool to learn of ways to protect their typically developing offspring from psychosocial difficulties.

REVIEW OF PAST RESEARCH ON PSYCHOSOCIAL FUNCTIONING IN SB
Research on Children and Adolescents

Previous studies have shown that youth with SB are at risk for exhibiting higher levels of internalizing symptoms (eg, depression, anxiety) and lower levels of self-concept than comparison children.[2,21,51,52] Those with hydrocephalus often exhibit difficulties in certain areas of cognitive functioning and school performance (eg, arithmetical, nonverbal cognitive skills[53];). Such children are also more likely to exhibit attention and concentration difficulties in school settings and tend to score at the low end of the average range of intelligence.[53–55]

To date, more work has been done in evaluating children with SB in the areas just noted than has been conducted in the area of social adjustment. This lack of attention is surprising given that this area of psychosocial functioning is problematic for most children with SB.[2,26] Youth with SB, compared with typically developing youth and those with other chronic conditions, tend to be socially immature and passive, to have fewer friends, to be less likely to have social contacts outside school, and to date less during adolescence,[2,26,56] and these difficulties seem to be maintained over time.[54]

The degree to which an adolescent exhibits decision-making autonomy in both medical and nonmedical areas is another highly salient developmentally oriented variable for these youth and their families.[57,58] Typically developing adolescents view more issues as falling within their own decision-making jurisdiction than they did during childhood and they are also increasingly likely to question the legitimacy of parental authority.[59–61] Holmbeck and colleagues'[2] findings on youth with SB run contrary to this typical developmental trend. Specifically, findings revealed that children and adolescents with SB (and especially boys and those with lower levels of intelligence) tend to be more dependent on adults for guidance, less likely to exhibit behavioral autonomy at home, less likely to exhibit intrinsic motivation at school, and less likely to express their own viewpoints during observed family interactions.[40,58,61] Variation in intrinsic motivation (ie, interest in learning and mastery, curiosity, preference for challenge) proved to be the most robust predictor of psychosocial adaptation (ie, scholastic success, social acceptance, and positive self-worth) in a study by Coakley and colleagues.[62]

Research on Emerging Adults

Emerging adulthood is a critical period in the life of older adolescents with SB[63] (First World Congress on SB Research and Care, March 2009, Orlando, FL, USA[64,65]). In general, many young adults with SB are capable of high levels of independent functioning across multiple domains but most have not been successful in fully engaging in the larger community of typically developing emerging adults.[66] In this section, we review findings related to many of the major milestones of emerging adulthood (ie, psychosocial adjustment, educational achievement, and employment and vocational outcomes).

Regarding psychosocial adjustment, emerging adults with SB, like their younger counterparts, are at risk for depressive symptoms and anxiety.[67,68] Regarding educational outcomes, emerging adults with SB are less likely to go to college (41%–49% of individuals with SB go to college vs 66% of typically developing youth[69–71]). With respect to vocational outcomes, recent studies report rates of full- or part-time employment ranging from 36% to 41% (MH Bellin and colleagues. Gender differences in self-management, community integration, and quality of life in transition-age individuals with spina bifida, unpublished manuscript, 2010),[71–73] which are significantly lower than those found in typically developing youth (ie, roughly 75%[70,71,74]) and in those with other chronic conditions (eg, asthma, cancer; 68% to 78%[72,75]).

Little is known about factors that predict whether or not an emerging adult with SB is able to go to college and become employed. Studies that have been conducted on individuals with SB have tended to focus only on demographic or medical severity predictors. For example, Liptak and colleagues[72] found that communication problems, difficulties with managing responsibilities, lower levels of parental education, and higher rates of parental unemployment were associated with poorer social, vocational, and educational transitions. Bellin and colleagues (Gender differences in self-management, community integration, and quality of life in transition-age individuals with spina bifida, unpublished manuscript, 2010) found that young adult men with SB were more likely to work than women, but that women were more likely to live independently. With respect to medical severity, Hetherington and colleagues[76] found that spinal lesion level and number of shunt revisions were related to employment outcome (with higher lesion levels and more shunt revisions being related to worse occupational outcome; Barf and colleagues[77] found similar results in the Netherlands.

In the absence of data, many have speculated about why young adults with SB are less likely to be successful in negotiating these emerging adulthood milestones. For example, some have described the complexities in managing real world responsibilities with a chronic physical condition, including transportation difficulties and issues related to accessibility.[68,77] Other explanations for these developmental delays focus on financial concerns (including lack of health insurance[78]), lack of job training and vocational rehabilitation services, restricted experiences with self-management,[79] employment discrimination, stigmas related to physical appearance, and a lack of autonomy-related socialization in early childhood.[68,80,81] Many of these issues are addressed with the Life Course Model Web site resource and such content is likely useful for families.

HOW THE LIFE COURSE MODEL WEB SITE INFORMS AND EMPOWERS FAMILIES

This section focuses on the 3 major domains of the Web site: health and self-management, social relationships, and education/employment. The content within each domain is based on the theories discussed earlier and the research findings just reviewed in the areas of family functioning, psychosocial adjustment, and the development of independent functioning. Each of the Web site domains is designed to provide families with readily accessible guidance in raising and caring for children with SB. The Web site (see article by Zabel in this issue) presents strategies that families can use to foster developmental achievements within each domain as children progress from childhood into emerging adulthood and beyond. At the site, searches can be performed either by topic (health/condition self-management, social/personal relationships, education/employment) or by age (preschool, school-age, adolescence, or young adulthood) and searches can be saved or printed for easy reference. The abilities of individuals with SB vary greatly, and cognitive and emotional developmental level rather than a specific age is important to consider when using the Web site. In addition to using this Web site, formal evaluations by psychologists, social workers, occupational therapists, vocational therapists, and other professionals can aid families in determining appropriate interventions.

HEALTH AND SELF-MANAGEMENT: HELPING YOUTH TO BECOME SELF-RELIANT

The primary goal of the health/self-management domain is to help youth become self-reliant in managing their SB. To achieve this goal, the health/self-management section of the Web site contains evidence-based information and resources on SB and anticipatory guidance for families to assist them in managing their children's SB.

The Web site content of this domain is designed to facilitate families' understanding and competencies in managing the long-term health care and special needs of their children. The health information, anticipatory guidance, and resources available on the Web site serve to inform families on the application of evidence-based strategies for their children that aim to foster an optimal state of health, prevent the occurrence of complications and secondary conditions resulting in adverse health consequences, promote the development of a positive body image, and cultivate the development of self-management skills that culminates ultimately in youth who become more self-reliant in managing their SB.

Six areas of specific health concerns for children with SB are covered, including mobility, skin integrity, sexuality, obesity prevention, bowel and bladder management, and condition management. Each of the 6 health areas of the health/self-management domain begins with the identification of developmental milestones, which represent appropriate expectations for the identified health need that is aligned with the child's developmental stage. For example, during the preschool period, developmental milestones regarding sexuality begin with body awareness and naming body parts. During the school-age and adolescent periods, the developmental milestones build on the initial foundation of sexuality learned during the preschool period toward achieving an understanding of themselves as sexual beings. By adulthood, the key milestones are the development of an intact sexual identity and an understanding of sexual relationships.

In terms of condition management, a preschooler's expected milestone achievement of SB knowledge is shown by the following 4 basic skills: (1) knows the name of SB and its functional effects on mobility and bowel and bladder management; (2) knows that SB is a long-term condition and is the reason for their functional limitations; (3) identifies medication by appearance; and (4) assists parent in ordering supplies and medications. The delineation of developmentally appropriate milestones in each of the 6 areas of health/self-management serves to inform parents concerning appropriate expectations for each developmental age.

Each key milestone is accompanied by descriptions of behaviors that the child/young person/young adult should show if they have achieved this milestone. For example, in the area of sexuality, the preschool child is expected to know the difference between good and bad touching, engage in gender-based imaginary role-playing, and be able to name the anatomic body parts on a doll. The descriptions of behaviors that indicate achievement of milestones in health/self-management provide families with concrete examples to evaluate their children's progress in meeting the developmental milestones. The extent to which the child achieves or fails to achieve developmental milestones in any of the 6 areas of the health/self-management domain creates opportunities for the family to consult with the specialized team and/or primary care pediatrician as part of the child's developmental surveillance during regularly scheduled specialty or primary care appointments.

The Web site offers specific ideas for interventions, resources, and referrals for each of the health/self-management areas. For example, recommendations to improve skin integrity for the school-age child include wearing seamless socks to reduce pressure on the feet, ensuring that the child does not walk in bare feet, washing and checking feet daily, and trimming toenails regularly. Further, these suggestions are coupled with a list of resources and referrals for families, including professionals who may be consulted, a specialty shoe retailer, and other Web sites for skin-care assistance.

The information in the health/self-management domain was developed to address families' concerns and uncertainties as to what are developmentally appropriate and reasonable expectations for their children. This Web site provides parents with evidence-based health information, guidance, and resources to inform and empower families to assist their child with SB in managing the condition.

SOCIAL RELATIONSHIPS: DEVELOPING A SOCIAL NETWORK

As noted earlier, individuals with SB have been reported to be less satisfied with partnership relations[82] when compared with peers who do not have SB, and to report low levels of social activities with peers.[66] Although factors that indicate greater severity or involvement of the condition, such as the presence of hydrocephalus, higher level of lesion, or the use of a wheelchair, have been correlated with less participation in society, even persons who are community ambulators have been found to score low on social integration measures.[68]

In light of these findings and the intuitive significance of relationships and participation in society, this domain of the Web site outlines developmental milestones from young childhood to young adulthood that are considered to increase the chances of developing fulfilling personal and social relationships throughout the life course. The development of relationships with parents, siblings, friends, and intimate/romantic partners was targeted during preschool, school-age, adolescence, and the young adulthood years, respectively. In addition, tips and interventions that may be helpful in the achievement of a particular age-specific milestone are offered to enhance preexisting strengths and address areas of concern.

As an example of how one might use this Web site, suppose that a mother of a preschool-aged child with SB is interested in learning more about how to help her child develop friendships. She can log on to the site, navigate to the preschool age category and, from there, navigate to the relationships domain. She is prompted to consider how her own child is developing in the area of making and keeping friends. Young children are not expected to have a flourishing social network but the information provided gives developmentally appropriate pointers regarding some of the milestones that parents can consider in the area of developing friendships. The Web site is intended as a resource and to complement, but not replace, professional opinion or assessment.

If the mother decides to learn more about how her child can develop more positive relations with his/her parents, she finds that a close attachment between child and parent is highlighted as a developmental milestone. In the corresponding tips and intervention section, information is available on secure attachment as well as some parenting strategies likely to increase the chances of achieving a secure attachment. A parent of a school-aged child with SB who is concerned with sibling relations might be prompted to look for warm relationships between siblings. This milestone references the initial development of empathy and the management of conflict. In addition, the need for the sibling of the child with SB to meet their own developmental needs is stressed. Examples of corresponding tips include points on bullying, problem solving, and conflict resolution, as well as the importance of focusing on the siblings' experiences and achievements. Relationships with friends are especially important during adolescence; thus, developmental milestones in this section emphasize the importance of having close, same- age/gender friends and that the adolescent participate in group activities with friends. If those milestones are met, there may be no need to delve into the tips available. However, if the milestones are not met, concrete information is available on strategies that can be used to increase the chances of making friends and participating in group activities.

Whereas the parents of a child with SB are the most likely family members to use the Web site during the younger developmental stages, the individual with SB may be the most likely candidate to search the adolescent or young adult sections pertaining to social relationships. For a young adult, relationships with intimate and romantic partners may be of interest. Milestones discussed include, for example, the preservation of self-esteem and self-confidence, the ongoing development of social coping strategies, and the development of assertiveness and social initiative. Some of the tips include strategies for engaging in social opportunities, steps to increase the likelihood of successful social interactions, and maintaining contact with a large group of friends even if the young person is already dating.

EDUCATION, EMPLOYMENT, AND INCOME SUPPORT: ACHIEVING THE MILESTONES OF EMERGING ADULTHOOD

Parenting involves preparing one's child to become an independent adult. As reviewed in previous sections, for parents of children with SB, this task is complicated by the medical, psychosocial, and neurocognitive difficulties associated with SB, such as a complex medical regimen, difficulties with ambulation and mobility, and problems with executive functions. Preparing one's child to achieve the developmental milestones of emerging adulthood begins as early as the preschool years, although the target skills and milestones vary as a function of the child's developmental level. Facilitating cognitive development and developmentally appropriate responsibility taking at an early age can set one's child on a trajectory for success in later years. The aim of this domain of the Web site is to allow parents to identify strengths and areas for improvement regarding education and employment based on their child's developmental level, and to build their child's competencies to promote future milestone achievement. The Web site resources may be particularly useful during times of transition, such as academic transitions (eg, from elementary school to middle school or high school) and vocational transitions (eg, preparing a teenager or young adult for their first job).

Preschool

Although preschool is a long way from emerging adulthood, early cognitive development helps set the foundation for later academic and vocational success. The Web site provides questions for parents to assess their child's achievement of important cognitive developmental milestones at this age, such as early object use, problem-solving skills, symbolic play, and visual perception. Developmentally appropriate responsibility-taking skills can also be evaluated, such as participating in feeding and dressing oneself and cleaning up after oneself. The assessment questions are not meant to be a substitute for a formal cognitive or developmental evaluation; however, these questions can be useful in identifying areas of strength and weakness and may indicate the need for a professional evaluation. The Web site also provides some general information and Web links regarding how to seek early intervention services, assessment tools often used by professionals, and important laws, such as the Individuals with Disabilities Education Act (IDEA). Furthermore, there are practical suggestions for parents to facilitate the development of specific skills or enhance strengths that children already show. For example, to encourage the development of decision-making skills, parents can provide children with age-appropriate choices, such as wearing a green or blue shirt, or drinking milk or juice. The Web site also provides references for further reading and links to helpful resources, including lists of developmentally appropriate toys.

School Age

The focus of the school-age years is on academic engagement and success, and increased participation in self-care and household chores. Assessment at this developmental stage examines academic success in fundamental subjects such as reading and mathematics, as well as whether the child is exhibiting core processing deficits associated with meningomyelocele, including executive function, memory, and attention problems. These deficits can negatively affect academic performance and the ability to follow through with responsibilities. Time-management skills also become increasingly important during the school-age years. The Web site suggests that parents seek a neuropsychological assessment for their child so that interventions, if needed, can be individually tailored to meet their child's needs. The Web site provides several practical suggestions for improving specific areas of weakness, such as functional mathematical skills, memory problems, and organizational skills. Parents may want to share some of the references and tools provided by the Web site with their child's teachers to assist the child in using such strategies in the school environment. Furthermore, the Web site informs parents that children are entitled to a free and appropriate public education and encourages parents to advocate for the most appropriate services for their child. The Web site also contains recommendations that parents set age-appropriate expectations for household responsibilities, such as regular chores, participating in self-care, caring for personal devices (eg, braces, wheelchair), getting ready for school, and managing an allowance. Recommendations regarding setting up routines and making environmental modifications, such as placing items needed to complete chores within reach, are provided to help parents assist their children in successfully increasing their responsibilities at home.

Adolescence

The Web site focuses on preparing adolescents for the transition into emerging and young adulthood, shifting from general cognitive development to vocational development. It is recommended that parents work with school personnel to develop a specific transition plan as part of their adolescent's Individualized Education Plan. An additional milestone of this age is to begin to explore meaningful and realistic career options. Parents can provide opportunities for exposure to various careers and post-secondary educational options, as well as help adolescents continue to develop the interpersonal and organizational skills that influence success in the workplace. Families can help teenagers identify areas of strength that can become a vocational pursuit and reward the teenager's efforts toward building skills in the chosen area. Although there is great variability among individuals, adolescence is generally characterized by increased responsibility for oneself and one's actions. Parents can help foster an adolescent's autonomy by teaching skills to care for oneself and one's personal belongings, including increased independence in medical self-management and hygiene. In addition, the Web site focuses on increasing responsibility outside the home through increased community engagement, navigation of the community through driving or public transportation, and volunteer or paid job experiences. The practical suggestions offered by the Web site may be helpful for both parents and teens.

Emerging Adulthood

All of the sections discussed thus far are geared toward helping a child achieve the milestones of emerging adulthood, including participating in postsecondary education or training for employment, beginning a career, obtaining financial security, sustaining health benefits, living independently, and balancing employment/personal life responsibilities. The information on the Web site aims to teach both young adults and their families to evaluate their success in achieving milestones and build skills to do so. The Web site gradually shifts the focus from the parent understanding their child's strengths and weaknesses to the young adult with SB increasing their self-awareness of individual strengths and weaknesses. Some assessment tools are referred to that may aid parents and adults in determining appropriate living situations. Parents are encouraged to assist their adult child in developing skills of self-evaluation, self-questioning, and self-checking, rather than problem solving for the adult. Parents may direct their adult children to this Web site for resources on how to solve some of the problems they encounter or use the Web site together to help the adult evaluate current strengths and choose an area of weakness for targeted behavior change.

SUMMARY

In this article, we have discussed how this developmentally oriented Life Course Model Web site can be useful for parents of youth with SB and for the youth themselves as they move toward the emerging adulthood stage of development. As with any intervention, the concern is that families who most need such support are also those who are the least likely to use this valuable resource. Thus, it is critical for the developers of the Life Course Model Web site to provide outreach to the most at-risk populations and to those who have limited access to computer resources. Because the Web site is developmentally oriented, parents and youth are able to make use of this site beginning in early childhood and across the various stages of child development, and young adults can make use of this tool as they transition to early adulthood. As has been done with similar Web-based resources developed for youth with other chronic health conditions,[6] evaluation should be conducted on the feasibility and usefulness of this resource for families and individuals affected by SB.

REFERENCES

1. Greenley RN, Holmbeck GN, Zukerman J, et al. Psychosocial adjustment and family relationships in children and adolescents with spina bifida. In: Wyszynski DF, editor. Neural tube defects: from origin to treatment. New York: Oxford University Press; 2006. p. 307–24.
2. Holmbeck GN, Westhoven VC, Phillips WS, et al. A multimethod, multi-informant, and multidimensional perspective on psychosocial adjustment in preadolescents with spina bifida. J Consult Clin Psychol 2003;71:782–95.
3. Kelly LM, Zebracki K, Holmbeck GN, et al. Adolescent development and family functioning in youth with spina bifida. J Pediatr Rehabil Med 2008;1:291–302.
4. Singh DK. Families of children with spina bifida: a review. J Dev Phys Disabil 2003;15:37–55.
5. Holmbeck GN, Greenley RN, Coakley RM, et al. Family functioning in children and adolescents with spina bifida: an evidence-based review of research and interventions. J Dev Behav Pediatr 2006;27:249–77.
6. Ritterband LM, Palermo TM. Introduction to the special issue: eHealth in pediatric psychology. J Pediatr Psychol 2009;34:453–6.
7. Long AC, Palermo TM. Brief report: web-based management of adolescent chronic pain: development and usability of an online family cognitive behavioral therapy program. J Pediatr Psychol 2009;34:511–6.
8. Lewis D. Computer-based approaches to patient education: a review of the literature. J Am Med Inform Assoc 1999;6:272–82.
9. Wade SL, Walz NC, Carey JC, et al. Brief report: description of feasibility and satisfaction findings from an innovative online family problem-solving intervention for adolescents following traumatic brain injury. J Pediatr Psychol 2009;34:517–22.
10. Ewing LJ, Long K, Rotondi A, et al. Brief report: a pilot study of a web-based resource for families of children with cancer. J Pediatr Psychol 2009;34:523–9.

11. Law M, Hanna S, King G, et al. Factors affecting family-centered service delivery for children with disabilities. Child Care Health Dev 2003;29:357–66.
12. Rosenbaum P, King S, Law M, et al. Family-centered service: a conceptual framework and research review. Phys Occup Ther Pediatr 1998;18:1–20.
13. Shelton T, Jeppson E, Johnson B. Family-centered care for children with special health care needs. Washington, DC: Association for the Care of Children's Health; 1987.
14. Moore MH, Mah JK, Trute B. Family-centred care and health-related quality of life of patients in paediatric neurosciences. Child Care Health Dev 2009;35: 454–61.
15. Nijhuis BJ, Reinders-Messelink HA, de Blecourt AC, et al. Family-centered care in family-specific teams. Clin Rehabil 2007;21:660–71.
16. Wagner EH. Chronic disease management: what will it take to improve care for chronic illness? Eff Clin Pract 1998;1:2–4.
17. Wagner EH, Austin BT, Davis C, et al. Improving chronic illness care: translating evidence into action. Health Aff 2001;20:64–78.
18. Glasgow RE, Wagner EH, Schaefer J, et al. Development and validation of the Patient Assessment of Chronic Illness Care (PACIC). Med Care 2005;43:436–44.
19. Wagner EH, Bennett SM, Austin BT, et al. Finding common ground: patient-centeredness and evidence-based chronic illness care. J Altern Complement Med 2005;11(S1):7–15.
20. Gall C, Kingsworth S, Healy H. Growing up ready: a shared management approach. Phys Occup Ther Pediatr 2006;26(4):47–56.
21. Ammerman RT, Kane VR, Slomka GT, et al. Psychiatric symptomatology and family functioning in children and adolescents with spina bifida. J Clin Psychol Med Settings 1998;5:449–65.
22. Costigan CL, Floyd FJ, Harter KSM, et al. Family process and adaptation to children with mental retardation: disruption and resilience in family problem-solving interactions. J Fam Psychol 1997;11:515–29.
23. Holmbeck GN, Coakley RM, Hommeyer JS, et al. Observed and perceived dyadic and systemic functioning in families of preadolescents with spina bifida. J Pediatr Psychol 2002;27:177.
24. Coakley RM, Holmbeck GN, Friedman D, et al. A longitudinal study of pubertal timing, parent-child conflict, and cohesion in families of young adolescents with spina bifida. J Pediatr Psychol 2002;27:461–73.
25. Jandasek B, Holmbeck GN, DeLucia C, et al. Trajectories of family processes across the adolescent transition in youth with spina bifida. J Fam Psychol 2009;23:726–38.
26. Blum RW, Resnick MD, Nelson R, et al. Family and peer issues among adolescents with SB and cerebral palsy. Pediatrics 1991;88:280–5.
27. Holmbeck GN, Gorey-Ferguson L, Hudson T, et al. Maternal, paternal, and marital functioning in families of preadolescents with spina bifida. J Pediatr Psychol 1997;22:167–81.
28. Kronenberger WG, Thompson RJ Jr. Medical stress, appraised stress, and the psychological adjustment of mothers of children with myelomeningocele. J Dev Behav Pediatr 1992;13:405–11.
29. Vermaes IPR, Janssens J, Bosman AMT, et al. Parents' psychological adjustment in families of children with spina bifida: a meta-analysis. BMC Pediatr 2005;5:32–44.
30. Macias MM, Saylor CF, Haire KB, et al. Predictors of paternal versus maternal stress in families of children with neural tube defects. Child Health Care 2007; 36:99–115.

31. Vermaes IPR, Gerris JRM, Janssens J. Parents' social adjustment in families of children with spina bifida: a theory-driven review. J Pediatr Psychol 2007;32: 1214–26.

32. Barakat LP, Linney JA. Optimism, appraisals, and coping in the adjustment of mothers and their children with spina bifida. J Child Fam Stud 1995;4:303–20.

33. Grosse SD, Flores AL, Ouyang L, et al. Impact of spina bifida on parental caregivers: findings from a survey of Arkansas families. J Child Fam Stud 2009;18:574–81.

34. Sawin KJ, Bellin MH, Roux G, et al. The experience of parenting an adolescent with spina bifida. Rehabil Nurs 2003;28:173–85.

35. Barakat LP, Linney JA. Children with physical handicaps and their mothers: the interrelation of social support, maternal adjustment, and child adjustment. J Pediatr Psychol 1992;17:725.

36. Fagan J, Schor D. Mothers of children with spina bifida: factors related to maternal psychosocial functioning. Am J Orthopsychiatry 1993;63:146–52.

37. Kronenberger WG, Thompson RJ Jr. Psychological adaptation of mothers of children with spina bifida: association with dimensions of social relationships. J Pediatr Psychol 1992;17:1–14.

38. Macias MM, Clifford SC, Saylor CF, et al. Predictors of parenting stress in families of children with spina bifida. Child Health Care 2001;30:57–65.

39. McKernon WL, Holmbeck GN, Colder CR, et al. Longitudinal study of observed and perceived family influences on problem-focused coping behaviors of preadolescents with spina bifida. J Pediatr Psychol 2001;26:41–54.

40. Holmbeck GN, Johnson SZ, Wills KE, et al. Observed and perceived parental overprotection in relation to psychosocial adjustment in preadolescents with a physical disability: the mediational role of behavioral autonomy. J Consult Clin Psychol 2002;70:96–110.

41. Holmbeck GN, Shapera WE, Hommeyer JS. Observed and perceived parenting behaviors and psychosocial adjustment in preadolescents with spina bifida. In: Barber BK, editor. Intrusive parenting: how psychological control affects children and adolescents. Washington, DC: American Psychological Association; 2002. p. 191–234.

42. Seefeldt T, Holmbeck GN, Belvedere MC, et al. Socioeconomic status and democratic parenting in families of preadolescents with spina bifida. Psi Chi Journal of Undergraduate Research 1997;2:5–12.

43. Tew B, Laurence KM. Mothers, brothers and sisters of patients with spina bifida. Dev Med Child Neurol 1973;15:69–76.

44. Kazak AE, Clark MW. Stress in families of children with myelomeningocele. Dev Med Child Neurol 1986;28:220–8.

45. Bellin MH, Kovacs PJ, Sawin KJ. Risk and protective influences in the lives of siblings of youths with spina bifida. Health Soc Work 2008;33:199–209.

46. Kiburz JA. Perceptions and concerns of the school-age siblings of children with myelomeningocele. Issues Compr Pediatr Nurs 1994;17:223–31.

47. Taylor V, Charman T, Fuggle P. Well sibling psychological adjustment to chronic physical disorder in a sibling: how important is maternal awareness of their illness attitudes and perceptions? J Child Psychol Psychiatry 2001;42:953–62.

48. Williams PD, Williams AR, Graff JC, et al. Interrelationships among variables affecting well siblings and mothers in families of children with a chronic illness or disability. J Behav Med 2002;25:411–24.

49. Williams PD, Williams AR, Hanson S, et al. Maternal mood, family functioning, and perceptions of social support, self-esteem, and mood among siblings of chronically ill children. Child Health Care 1999;28:297–310.

50. Bellin MH, Bentley KJ, Sawin KJ, et al. Factors associated with the psychological and behavioral adjustment of siblings of youths with spina bifida. Fam Syst Health 2009;27:1–15.

51. Appleton PL, Elis NC, Minchom PE, et al. Depressive symptoms and self-concept in young people with spina bifida. J Pediatr Psychol 1997;22:707.

52. Shields N, Taylor NF, Dodd KJ. Self-concept in children with spina bifida compared with typically developing children. Dev Med Child Neurol 2008;50: 733–43.

53. Fletcher JM, Dennis M. Spina bifida and hydrocephalus. In: Yeates KO, Ris MD, Taylor HG, et al, editors. Pediatric neuropsychology: research, theory, and practice. 2nd edition. New York: Guilford; 2010. p. 3–25.

54. Holmbeck GN, DeLucia C, Essner B, et al. Trajectories of psychosocial adjustment in adolescents with spina bifida: a six-year four-wave longitudinal follow-up. J Consult Clin Psychol 2010;78:511–25.

55. Hommeyer JS, Holmbeck GN, Wills KE, et al. Condition severity and psychosocial functioning in pre-adolescents with spina bifida: disentangling proximal functional status and distal adjustment outcomes. J Pediatr Psychol 1999;24:409–509.

56. Ellerton ML, Stewart MJ, Ritchie JA, et al. Social support in children with a chronic condition. Can J Nurs Res 1996;28:15.

57. Anderson BJ, Coyne JC. Family context and compliance behavior in chronically ill children. In: Krasnegor NA, Epstein L, Johnson SB, et al, editors. Developmental aspects of health compliance behavior. Hillsdale (NJ): Erlbaum; 1993. p. 77–89.

58. Friedman D, Holmbeck GN, DeLucia C, et al. Trajectories of autonomy development across the adolescent transition in children with spina bifida. Rehabil Psychol 2009;54:16–27.

59. Darling N, Cumsille P, Martinez ML. Individual differences in adolescents' beliefs about the legitimacy of parental authority and their own obligation to obey: a longitudinal investigation. Child Dev 2008;79:1103–18.

60. Smetana JG. Concepts of self and social convention: adolescents' and parents' reasoning about hypothetical and actual family conflicts. Development during the transition to adolescence. In: Gunnar MR, Collins WA, editors, Minnesota symposia of child psychology, vol. 21. Hillsdale (NJ): Erlbaum; 1988. p. 79–122.

61. Davis BE, Shurtleff DB, Walker WO, et al. Acquisition of autonomy skills in adolescents with myelomeningocele. Dev Med Child Neurol 2006;48:253–8.

62. Coakley RM, Holmbeck GN, Bryant FB. Constructing a prospective model of psychosocial adaptation in young adolescents with spina bifida: an application of optimal data analysis. J Pediatr Psychol 2006;31:1084–99.

63. Blum R, Hirsch D, Kastner TA, et al. A consensus statement on health care transitions for young adults with special health care needs. Pediatrics 2002;110: 1304–6.

64. Holmbeck GN, Bauman L, Essner B, et al. Developmental context: the transition from adolescence to emerging adulthood in youth with disabilities and chronic health conditions. In: Lollar D, editor. Launching into adulthood: an integrated response to support transition of youth with chronic health conditions and disabilities. Baltimore (MD): Brookes; 2010. p. 21–47.

65. Lollar D, editor. The transition to adulthood in youth with disabilities and chronic health conditions. Baltimore (MD): Brookes; 2010.

66. Buran CF, Sawin KJ, Brei TJ, et al. Adolescents with myelomeningocele: activities, beliefs, expectations, and perceptions. Dev Med Child Neurol 2004;46:244–52.

67. Bellin MH, Zabel TA, Dicianno BE, et al. Correlates of depressive and anxiety symptoms in young adults with spina bifida. J Pediatr Psychol 2010;35:778–89.

68. Dicianno BE, Gaines A, Collins DM, et al. Mobility, assistive technology use, and social integration among adults with spina bifida. Am J Phys Med Rehabil 2009; 88:533.

69. Bowman RM, McLone DG, Grant JA, et al. Spina bifida outcome: a 25-year prospective. Pediatr Neurosurg 2000;34:114–20.

70. Cohen P, Kasen S, Chen H, et al. Variations in patterns of developmental transitions in the emerging adulthood period. Dev Psychol 2003;39:657–68.

71. Zukerman JM, Devine KA, Holmbeck GN. Adolescent predictors of emerging adult milestones in youth with spina bifida: a longitudinal study. J Pediatr Psychol, in press.

72. Liptak GS, Kennedy JA, Dosa NP. Youth with spina bifida and transitions: using the WHO ICF model in a nationally representative sample. Orlando (FL): First World Congress on Spina Bifida Research and Care; March, 2009.

73. McDonnell GV, McCann JP. Link between the CSF shunt and achievement in adults with spina bifida. J Neurol Neurosurg Psychiatry 2000;68:800.

74. Hamilton SF, Hamilton MA. School, work, and emerging adulthood. In: Arnett JJ, Tanner JL, editors. Emerging adults in America: coming of age in the 21st century. Washington, DC: American Psychological Association; 2006. p. 257–77.

75. Gerhardt CA, Dixon M, Miller K, et al. Educational and occupational outcomes among survivors of childhood cancer during the transition to emerging adulthood. J Dev Behav Pediatr 2007;28:448.

76. Hetherington R, Dennis M, Barnes M, et al. Functional outcome in young adults with spina bifida and hydrocephalus. Childs Nerv Syst 2006;22:117–24.

77. Barf HA, Post MWM, Verhoef M, et al. Restrictions in social participation of young adults with spina bifida. Disabil Rehabil 2009;31:921–7.

78. Park MJ, Mulye TP, Adams SH, et al. The health status of young adults in the United States. J Adolesc Health 2006;39:305–17.

79. Sawin KJ, Bellin MH, Roux G, et al. The experience of self-management in adolescent women with spina bifida. Rehabil Nurs 2009;34:26–38.

80. Dicianno BE, Kurowski BG, Yang JMJ, et al. Rehabilitation and medical management of the adult with spina bifida. Am J Phys Med Rehabil 2008;87:1027.

81. Schriner KF, Roessler RT, Johnson P. Identifying the employment concerns of people with spina bifida. J Appl Rehabil Counsel 1993;24:32.

82. Barf HA, Post MW, Verhoef M, et al. Life satisfaction of young adults with spina bifida. Dev Med Child Neurol 2007;49:458–63.

Spina Bifida: What We Learned from Consumers

Cecily L. Betz, PhD, RN[a,b,]*, Ronna Linroth, PhD, OT[c],
Carley Butler, ACSW[b], Jill Caruso, Amy Colgan-Niemeyer, CPT, CES,
Jamie Smith

KEYWORDS

- Spina bifida • Spina bifida consumer • Health care transitions
- Spina bifida personal experience

In the professional literature, much is written about the causative factors associated with spina bifida, its prevention, and the interdisciplinary approaches to addressing the biopsychosocial needs for treatment.[1–4] From the consumer perspective, for those who have spina bifida, the operative word about the knowledge and science of spina bifida is "about." That is, the literature to inform constituent groups, whether they are interdisciplinary professionals, policymakers, advocates, parents, or individuals with spina bifida themselves, often "lacks the voice" of those who live with spina bifida every moment of their lives.

The advances in medical treatment and interdisciplinary management of spina bifida have led to impressive improvements in the life expectancy of individuals with spina bifida. Issues of survival recede as quality of life issues and concerns about adulthood potential draw greater attention.[5] As has been discussed throughout this issue, comprehensive preparation for adulthood, beginning in early childhood, is of vital importance to foster the attainment of the lifetime goals that individuals with spina bifida dream and seek to achieve.

Best and evidence-based practices are predicated on data gathered through empiric means, expert practice, and the wisdom and insights of others who have had the lived experience, whether the consumers themselves or their family members. This article provides the perspectives and insights of several individuals with spina bifida who have experienced the transition experience themselves. Their unvarnished

[a] Department of Pediatrics, Keck School of Medicine, University of Southern California, 5000 Sunset Boulevard, Los Angeles, CA 90027, USA
[b] USC Center of Excellence in Developmental Disabilities, Children's Hospital Los Angeles, 4650 Sunset Boulevard, MS# 53, Los Angeles, CA 90027, USA
[c] Adult Outpatient Services, Gillette Children's Specialty Healthcare, St Paul, MN, USA
* Corresponding author. Department of Pediatrics, Keck School of Medicine, University of Southern California, Los Angeles, CA.
E-mail address: CLBetz@aol.com

Pediatr Clin N Am 57 (2010) 935–944
doi:10.1016/j.pcl.2010.07.013
0031-3955/10/$ – see front matter © 2010 Elsevier Inc. All rights reserved.

stories will open the door, metaphorically speaking, to their own candid reflections of this important period of time in their lives. These personal commentaries, each one unique, reveal the commonalities of this shared life experience. Next, preliminary findings of a longitudinal study entitled, "Examining the Trajectory of Transition in Adolescents and Young Adults with Spina Bifida," conducted at the Gillette Lifetime Specialty Healthcare Clinic, is presented. The compilation of personal impressions serves to inform those involved in the provision of care, services, policymaking, and advocacy services to youth and young adults with spina bifida, their families, and their circle of support of what is of foremost importance during this period of transition. The article concludes with recommendations, many of which can be located in the new transition Web-based resource, for the provision of youth- and adult-centered services and resources.

AMY'S STORY

Amy's reflections about living and growing up as a child with spina bifida and later as an adolescent and young adult, reveal a number of significant influences and challenges she faced. As Amy tells her story, she recounts the very important role her parents had in her life—a role of support and guidance, which at times she described as "overprotective." Her description of her school experiences in high school and college reveal the challenges that she encountered without the assistance of comprehensive transition planning, including for health care planning. Today, experts and advocates alike recognize the importance of supporting families and children with complex medical conditions, including spina bifida, to access services and/or programs that will assist children to develop self-advocacy and self-determination skills as exemplified with the development of the life span Web-based resource tool.[6,7] Amy's brief autobiography reveals the power of her positive and accepting attitude toward living her life to its fullest. The following is Amy's story.

There are many factors that affect how we handle life transitions, but to me the most significant one is the family. Mine has always been supportive. My parents made sure I got the care I needed. But I was also overly protected. Their concentration, understandably, was on doing all they could to help me survive and walk rather than encouraging independence. Yet I've struggled with confidence issues throughout my life, which I believe stem in part from that protectiveness. It is vital, in my opinion, for children with spina bifida to be encouraged to explore their world and be independent.

I was excited to enter the new world of school that my older siblings got to experience every day. I was mainstreamed, which I think was a good idea, but I became aware that I was different from the other kids, some of whom stared and made fun of my wobble walk. School took me out of my comfort zone. My self-consciousness grew. I believe now that counseling could have helped but, to my knowledge, it wasn't suggested by my medical team.

For health reasons, I was frequently absent from class and found it increasingly difficult to keep up with my work. The teachers and staff, although generally caring, didn't seem to know how to handle my situation. Early on, I went to physical education classes but spent most of the time on the sidelines. No arrangements were made for activities specific to my capabilities, and eventually I was exempt from physical education classes altogether. And I was held back in second grade because of frequent absenteeism more than an inability to do the work. After a rough start, the school provided more tutoring to help me keep up. I preferred this one-on-one learning experience over being in a classroom full of other kids.

With the help of family, friends, understanding teachers, and counseling, I blossomed in high school. My health improved, as did my confidence. I joined clubs, attended school dances, and did volunteer work. But I was still exempt from physical education classes. The school nurse tried to arrange something for me, but by then, unfortunately, I wasn't interested. I had too often gotten out of doing what I didn't want to, and I remained stubborn.

That stubbornness led me to go away to college. But it backfired. I was living 6 hours from home, confronted with responsibilities I was ill-prepared to face on my own—most notably health maintenance. I quit after 2 weeks and entered the local community college the next year, where I thrived. There, I was required to take an activity class, so I chose Personal Fitness. The teacher was understanding toward my limitations and adjusted workouts accordingly. It was one of my favorite classes. I also worked as a tutor in my spare time.

Throughout my adult life, I've fought depression, confidence issues, and preconceived notions of others. I let others think for me quite often. But through growth and maturity, that attitude has slowly changed. I've explored different career paths. When one didn't work out, I tried something else. Through my experience with spina bifida, I've learned the importance of patience, health maintenance, and having empathy for others.

Transitions are a part of life. With a good base of support and a positive attitude, those with spina bifida can more smoothly navigate life transitions.

CARLEY'S STORY

As Carley relates in her report of the transition from adolescence to emerging adulthood, she acknowledges the helpful support she received from educators and other professionals to prepare for the transition to college and the world of work. Yet, this same level of assistance was not available from the team of health care professionals who managed her care for many years. Carley described her health care transition planning and transfer to adult health care as a "non-story," meaning that she did not receive the assistance she obviously needed.

Carley's disappointment with the lack of acknowledgment of the important milestone of the termination of her pediatric care is apparent as she describes "there was no fanfare," a ceremonial oversight by her pediatric providers. Curiously, this "rite of passage," an important one for both the recipient and provider of care is rarely, if ever, acknowledged. As one expert recommended, "Celebrate transitions as they occur with graduation ceremonies, certificates of completion, and other rites of passage."[8(p1313)] The lack of assistance with the transfer of her care from pediatric to adult providers is obvious as well. Instead, without the helpful guidance from a member of her longstanding specialized pediatric team, Carley forged ahead to locate her own adult physician. Carley's story follows.

In reflecting on my transition from pediatric to adult health care, I have trouble putting the experience into words. I realize that this is because, while I can clearly recall much preparation going into other transitions in my life, from high school to college and from college into the work force, I see my health care transition as a non-story, with few details to recall. In my educational and career transitions, I remember a lot of preparation, with teams of professionals coming together with me and possibly my parents, and discussing in detail what the next steps would be to help me reach my goals. For my health care transition, there was no fanfare, no official meetings where the next steps would be neatly spelled out to carry me on my way to my goal of optimal health care. I remember mention of final appointments with my pediatric doctors; however, there was no clear answer as to where I would go next for care. I was left to search through multiple provider lists from my mother's insurance carrier, hoping to find doctors who had at least a basic knowledge of spina bifida. Luckily, I have found doctors that I am confident will help me reach my health care goals; however, I know not everyone has the access to or knowledge of the health care system to navigate it as successfully as I have, which is why comprehensive health care transition planning is crucial for every adolescent with a chronic illness.

JAMIE'S STORY

As with Amy, Jamie's parents had an important role in her life. She credits her parents with not only supporting her but actively encouraging her to learn to become more self-determined and to learn to advocate for herself. She acknowledges her parents' efforts to foster self-management of her spina bifida in all aspects of her special health care needs from doing her own self-care to making her own decisions regarding her medical care. Her parents started early, apparently recognizing that learning to become independent involves a life span approach. In most schools, formalized transition begins between 14 and 16 years of age. Waiting until then to address transition issues can hinder development of these maturity milestones.[7,9,10] This same philosophic approach guided the development efforts of the Web-based resource. The following is Jamie's story.

When I consider transitioning into adult health care in regard to managing spina bifida, it's hard to pinpoint just when that happened. I think it's because, really, there were multiple steps to that transition.

I was blessed to have parents who knew I would be most successful if I was taught to be independent. I wasn't treated as their "disabled child," I was simply taught to manage my disability. What I mean is, I was treated like my able-bodied brother was with regard to expectations of responsibility, and so forth.

Another blessing was that my parents included me in on decisions about my medical care from an early age. This included treatment, but mostly on choosing doctors. I remember meeting a new neurosurgeon and I didn't like how he treated me (he spoke to my parents—not me, etc) so we never went back. I also was allowed to stop seeing my (wonderful) male pediatrician when I was 9 years old because I had started to develop "lady issues" that I felt a woman doctor should hear. So, I started seeing a "grown-up doctor" for my "grown-up issues." Through these experiences, I was being trained to gauge what kind of doctors I liked and thought were good for me.

I was also taught to make my own doctors' appointments from the time I was a young teenager. This is a vital skill that I don't understand waiting until adulthood to learn. Being able to know what doctors to call and when, as well as being able to articulate the reason for the visit is really not as hard as some people with spina bifida make it out to be, in all honesty. It's a simple phone call that is no more difficult or complicated than ordering a pizza.

All of these skills were incredibly important (and put to the test) when I left home to attend college 2 states away. I was dealing with doctors in a small town that didn't always fully understand the issues related to being an adult with spina bifida. I learned even better self-advocacy skills that I continue to practice more than a decade later.

What I continue to find challenging is knowing what issues I need to be aware of now that I'm an adult with spina bifida. I have the health care guide for adults, but there's been several times that I've been told that some of the tests mentioned in that book are not necessary. As there is only a growing amount of knowledge of adults with spina bifida, I never know if I should trust information from the Spina Bifida Association, or from doctors who are sitting right in front of me. This is where my decision skills come into play. I'm learning to gauge when I should fight for certain things or trust the doctor's judgment. It's a fine line that seems to continue moving.

One thing about this journey into adulthood is that it's not over yet. And that's not just because I have spina bifida. As I get older, there will be more and better treatments, but there will also be more issues. I believe I've been equipped with the latent skills to handle those as they arise.

JILL'S STORY

Jill's recollection of her childhood experiences in dealing with health care professionals demonstrate the absence of her "voice" in dealing with her medical condition. This lack of self-advocacy and self-determination carried over into the school setting as well, leaving Jill feeling uncomfortable in offering her preferences about what she wanted. As a result, Jill did not receive the instruction needed to thoroughly manage her spina bifida. Confidence in important skills such as recognizing the triggers for possible complications and illnesses and learning to become an informed consumer by adopting the practice of compiling her health care records for later use were undeveloped.[7,11] The lack of transition preparation is the same theme echoed in the recalled memories of Amy and Carley. The following is Jill's story.

When you are young, you are told to be seen and not heard. These are words that ring in my ears today. Although I believe in respecting your elders, I wish I would have listened to myself a little more. When doctors would talk they would always talk to my mom. I felt as if I weren't even in the room. The same thing happened when I was at school and had an IEP (Individual Educational Plan) meeting. The teacher would talk to my mom. I previously wondered, "Is this my health and education they are talking about?" This has came back to haunt me, not knowing or understanding what was going on.

Doctors would make predictions on my life expectancy; they actually said I would die at the age of 9. I'm here today to tell you I am now 44 years young with 2 beautiful children. Having children is something else doctors said would probably not happen. Most of these doctors have passed on or have retired; I wish they could see me today. I graduated from high school, attended college, and have been working since the age of 13. When I turned 18, I could no longer go to the Myelo Clinic because I was too old. I searched high and low for an adult clinic, but no such luck. After all, doctors didn't think individuals with spina bifida would reach the age of 18.

I then got wrapped up in my own life and forgot that I had a disability that may need medical attention and ongoing assessments. I waited until my body would hurt or my skin would break down before I sought out any medical help. Over and over they would say, "Why have you waited so long to get medical attention?" In my eyes, if it weren't broken, you didn't need to fix it. I feel now that if I had been more involved in my care as a teenager, I would be more proactive with my health care needs today.

In closing, if I could give any advice, it would be that you are your best advocate. Let your voice be heard. Please get involved in your medical care and your education. After all, it is your life and you only get one chance at it. Ask for copies of your medical records because I've been told that records are destroyed after 7 years. I can tell you this is true from my experience. I called the hospital where I had undergone several surgeries as a child, and I was told there are no records of any surgeries or treatments.

This is crucial because other physicians will not want to treat you if they don't know what procedures have been done in the past.

Each of these personal recollections reflects the need for ongoing support and assistance in learning the skills and knowledge needed to function independently and enjoy an improved quality of life. The reflections also reveal the importance of a sustained and ongoing life course approach to fostering the development of developmental competencies for individuals with spina bifida to realize their lifetime goals and dreams for the future.[7]

The next portion of this article reports insights learned from youth and young adults about their lifestyle experiences in living with spina bifida. Their candid sharing of information about their lives provides greater understanding of the challenges they have and continue to face as well as the achievements they have attained. These insights provide a view of their life experiences that serve to provide health care professionals with a unique form of evidence for practice purposes.

INSIGHTS FROM THE TRANSITION EXPERIENCES OF MINNESOTA YOUTH

Researchers at Gillette Lifetime Specialty Healthcare Clinic in St Paul, Minnesota, have been conducting the first and second of 3 annual interviews with youth in transition for a research study entitled, "Examining the Trajectory of Transition in Adolescents and Young Adults with Spina Bifida" (University of Minnesota IRB 0802S273241). In this recent series of interviews, youth described their transition journeys. Most could describe their disability in general terms, could give a basic health history, and tell what their medications were for, even if they were unable to name them. Several young adults described being independent with their own physical self-care but they continued to be dependent on parents for all other aspects of their special needs management; however, they indicated that they were generally satisfied with these circumstances.

When youth were asked to describe the nature of their social relationships, they revealed a variety of different types. The continuum of their personal relationships ranged from social isolation or relationships limited to family members or caregivers, to active electronic communication, but scant face-to-face interactions with a few close friends to the rare experience of actually socializing with small groups of friends in the community.

The section that follows presents excerpts from the interviews that illustrate some of the common themes from this research investigation. These themes are

- Challenges in preparation for self-management
- Limited social relationships
- Awareness of cognitive challenges
- Cost of independence.

The themes gathered from this study mirror many of the issues raised in the personal reflections written earlier.

Challenges in Preparation for Self-Management

When asked what percentage of their own care the youth preformed and what percentage their parents performed, one young woman replied, "I do 100% of my self-care and my mother does the administrative stuff." When pressed for detail, the young woman explained that she took care of her personal hygiene, dressed and fed herself, and had assigned household chores like doing the laundry, emptying the dishwasher, or caring for a pet. The caregiving activities performed by her mother, which she referred to as "administrative stuff" were dealing with paperwork, tasks that related to dealing with doctors, addressing insurance issues, ordering supplies, paying bills, and managing aspects of the youth's health condition. Following this clarification, the youth was once again asked what percentage she felt she was responsible for and what percentage her mother did, she replied, "I do 100% of what I do and she does 100% of what she does."

Some youth indicated an awareness of a need to adapt to new circumstances as they matured into adulthood. Most showed a general or vague concern about needing to learn more about managing their own affairs. For example, when discussing a young adult's understanding of his or her health insurance plan, their responses typified the attitude of not seriously attending to it, as evidenced by the statement, "I just worry about it when I have to." Instead, youth expressed a general awareness of the name of their health insurance plan but were unfamiliar with the details of their insurance plan coverage such as benefits available, copayment requirements, and the use of the appeal process in the event of a denial of services.

Some youth express a "stubbornness" about trying to do as much as they can for themselves, whereas others indicated an acceptance or desire to have someone else manage or comanage their lives. As one youth stated, "I'm not able to remember all my medications, so I'm always going to have to have somebody set them up for me."

Strategies for money management were limited. These strategies included asking their parents for funds when out of money and performing household jobs for neighbors like watering plants or pet sitting to earn a little cash. Others indicated that they were learning about using an ATM or managing a checking account. A few young people indicated that they were unable to balance their bank accounts; instead, they relied on calling the bank to obtain information about their balance. For them, it was a convenient strategy to determine the amount of money available to spend.

In contrast, one young man reported his money management had improved over the previous year. He said he used to forget to check his account balance via his bank's automated system before going out. However, negative consequences from that experience helped him learn to remember. As he remarked, "I'm a hands on learner. I can't learn by demonstration of others."

The study participants also reported having a range of household responsibilities. A few youth remarked that they were not required to perform household chores, whereas others reported having clear expectations of doing their "share" within the family and were treated no differently than their siblings. In addition, some indicated that beginning in their teens, they were responsible for ordering their medical supplies and making medical or transportation appointments.

Limited Social Relationships

Youth expressed feelings of social isolation from peers in postsecondary life with a dependence on family members for both planning and accompaniment in social activities. One young woman revealed the following insight about "fitting into" different social groups.

"I did not participate in diversity at my high school, and I do not plan to in college. In the past, I have had experiences where it appears to me that diversity starts working backward; [diversity groups] start creating more discrimination, although the result is positive. What ends up happening is that people start saying, 'Hey, I am going to become your friend because you're different' versus the equality that it is suppose to be promoting, which is you're my friend because you are another human being and we connect on this."

One young man indicated that he had never been alone by himself. At school, he typically had a friend accompany him on the elevator in the event it got stuck between floors. His explanation was, "Cause she's got a cell phone and I do too in case her cell phone dies, I can call for help." By age 18, he could still not think of a situation where he might be comfortable being alone out in the community if he had the opportunity to do so.

Some youth reported changing their self-catheterization schedule as well as altering or disbanding their taking of medications so as not to call attention to their differences when with others. In one situation, both the young woman being interviewed and her brother had a disability. She revealed that when they infrequently visited people, they "didn't feel comfortable" to have them see her and her brother with medications.

A sensitivity to appearing different from their peers or even extended family members resulted in neglect of self-care for some. This sensitivity to how others perceive them may explain the reluctance to use assistive technology or techniques that set them apart. That said, many in this group demonstrated a quick and ready adoption of technologies used to socialize. Perhaps because of the challenges of physically getting together with others, electronic communication networking through Facebook, Twitter, texting, and cell phones was popular. Although some used the technology for socializing, others had mastered the use of alarms, calendars, directions for finding their way, and preprogrammed phone books to augment their memory.

Awareness of Cognitive Challenges

Some youth with spina bifida were aware that they might hold a slightly different world view. They reported a reliance on verbal communication skills for navigating through situations, as they experienced difficulties with executive functioning, math, and reading comprehension. As one respondent stated, "I know how to be assertive. I think a weakness would be trying to verbalize kind of complex ideas. Sometimes I think I just see things a little bit different from some people." Another challenge identified by youth was associated with time. As one young man stated, "I will think that 2 hours has gone by and it is like 4 or 5 hours has gone by." When asked if the young man had adopted a strategy for tracking time, he said that people just reminded him of the time.

This young man reported he was aware of "cognitive problems such as having trouble getting thoughts out, learning disabilities, and difficulty with problem solving. He stated that he knows he is good "with verbal" and "not good with subtle hints." He summarized his abilities by revealing, "I have a hard time communicating my needs. I am not in tune with my own body and my own mind."

Way finding is another challenge encountered. Several youth talked about their concern for traveling alone. They were reluctant going alone to some place new or far away requiring additional efforts for travel. They were comfortable traveling alone to familiar places or those that were nearby.

Cost of Independence

Youth talked of their ambivalence in attempting to balance between their need for independence and their family. One young woman who had lived outside of the family home successfully, returned home primarily for financial reasons. Although she could make her living expenses, she did not have funds for discretionary spending. The young woman noted how her father had resumed "taking care" of her after she had moved back home. He shopped, cooked, cleaned, laundered the clothes, and basically did everything for her. He drove her to all of her medical appointments even though she had a car and driver's license. Although she wished for her lost independence, she was reluctant to negotiate with her father because she didn't want to hurt his feelings.

Another young woman who lived at home and whose supplemental security income contributed to the household expenses and grocery purchases, indicated that it was a good experience to know there was someone for her if she needed her parents. However, she has remained dependent on her parents and in effect has become reluctant to venture into the community and get engaged with outside activities. Her recognition of this problem, prompted her to say, "There are days where I've started to wonder what life would be if I lived on my own and had friends."

One young man in the study indicated that he did not want to be in charge of managing his health care saying it required too much effort. In effect, he allows others to decide when he should see doctors; although, when he has a health problem or need for medical supplies, he will inform the staff at the group home. His dependence on others for medically related needs is in stark contrast to other areas of his life as he stated, "They [group home staff] are responsible for probably 97% of my medical life. I'm in charge of 98% of my social and everything else." Just a year later, he indicated he was less satisfied with this arrangement.

In the course of these interviews it became evident that youth with spina bifida had opinions and experiences that were powerfully informative about how they perceive their place in the world. As this study has evolved, the respondents have become more self-disclosing with their responses. Our ability to probe more deeply has provided rich data for analysis.

RECOMMENDATIONS

As the "voices" of youth and adults with spina bifida have illustrated, living with a medically complex disability is difficult. However, this life journey can be made more manageable and meaningful with providing families from the very beginning with the access to services and supports to foster the development of their children's skill building in all life domains. The Life Course Model Web site described in other articles in this issue was designed to provide families with the resources to facilitate their efforts in this regard in these life domains: health self-management, personal-social relationships, employment, and income support.

This discussion raises the issue of how to accept reliance on others while maintaining a comfortable amount of independence.[12] Given the consumers' remarks about how much effort it takes for them to perform tasks independently, consumers, families, and care providers should strive to strike a balance between the benefits associated with independent task performance and the costs in time, effort, and personal stress.

REFERENCES

1. Bartonek A, Saraste H. Factors influencing ambulation in myelomeningocele: a cross-sectional study. Dev Med Child Neurol 2001;43(4):253–60.
2. Barf HA, Verhoef M, Jennekens-Schinkel A, et al. Cognitive status of young adults with spina bifida. Dev Med Child Neurol 2003;45(12):813–20.
3. Barf HA, Verhoef M, Post MW, et al. Educational career and predictors of type of education in young adults with spina bifida. Int J Rehabil Res 2004;27(1):45–52.
4. Bouilet SL, Gambrell D, Shin M, et al. Racial/ethnic differences in the birth prevalence of spina bifida: United States, 1995-2005. J Am Med Assoc 2009;301(21): 2203–4.

5. Thompson DNP. Postnatal management and outcome for neural tube defects including spina bifida and encephalocoeles. Prenat Diagn 2009;29(4):412–9.

6. Betz CL. Transition of adolescents with special health care needs: review and analysis of the literature. Issues Compr Pediatr Nurs 2004;27:179–240.

7. Betz CLN, Nehring WM. Promoting health care transition planning for adolescents with special health care needs and disabilities. Towson (MD): Brookes Publishing; 2007.

8. Reiss J, Gibson R. Health care transition: destinations unknown. Pediatrics 2002; 110(6 Pt 2):1307–14.

9. Nehring WM, Faux SA. Transitional and health issues of adults with neural tube defects. J Nurs Scholarsh 2006;38(1):63–70.

10. Roebroeck ME, Jahnsen R, Carona C, et al. Adult outcomes and lifespan issues for people with childhood-onset physical disability. Dev Med Child Neurol 2009; 51(8):670–8.

11. Betz CL, Redcay G, Tan S. Self-reported health care self-care needs of transition-aged youth: a pilot study. Issues Compr Pediatr Nurs 2003;26(3):159–81.

12. Stewart D, Freeman M, Law M, et al. "The Best Journey to Adult Life" for youth with disabilities: an evidence-based model and best practice guidelines for the transition to adulthood for youth with disabilities. In: CanChild Centre for Childhood Disability Research. Canada (ON): Institute for Applied Health Sciences, McMaster University; 2009.

Using the Spina Bifida Life Course Model in Clinical Practice: An Interdisciplinary Approach

Brad E. Dicianno, MD[a,b,*], Andrea D. Fairman, MOT, OTR/L, CPRP[c,d],
Shannon B. Juengst, MS, CRC[e],
Patricia G. Braun, DNSc, MSN, MA, CPNP, RNC[f],
T. Andrew Zabel, PhD, ABPP[g,h]

KEYWORDS

• Spina bifida • Development • Milestones • Transition

This work was supported by the National Spina Bifida Program, National Center on Birth Defects and Developmental Disabilities, Centers for Disease Control and Prevention, Atlanta, Georgia.

[a] Department of Veterans Affairs, Human Engineering Research Laboratories (HERL), VA Pittsburgh Healthcare System, 7180 Highland Drive, 151R-1, Pittsburgh, PA 15206, USA
[b] Adult Spina Bifida Clinic, Department of Physical Medicine and Rehabilitation, University of Pittsburgh Medical Center (UPMC), Kaufmann Medical Building, Suite 202, 3471 5th Avenue, Pittsburgh, PA 15213, USA
[c] Department of Rehabilitation Science and Technology, University of Pittsburgh, School of Health and Rehabilitation Sciences, Forbes Tower, Suite 5044, 3600 Forbes Avenue, Pittsburgh, PA 15260, USA
[d] Department of Physical Medicine and Rehabilitation, Adult Spina Bifida Clinic, University of Pittsburgh Medical Center (UPMC), Kaufmann Medical Building, Suite 202, 3471 5th Avenue, Pittsburgh, PA 15213, USA
[e] Department of Occupational Therapy, University of Pittsburgh, School of Health and Rehabilitation Sciences, Forbes Tower, Suite 5012, 3600 Forbes Avenue, Pittsburgh, PA 15260, USA
[f] School of Nursing and Health Studies, Northern Illinois University, 1240 Normal Road, DeKalb, IL 60115, USA
[g] Department of Neuropsychology, Philip A. Keelty Center for Spina Bifida and Related Conditions, Kennedy Krieger Institute, 1750 East Fairmount Avenue, Baltimore, MD 21231, USA
[h] Department of Psychiatry and Behavioral Sciences, Johns Hopkins University School of Medicine, 733 North Broadway, Baltimore, MD 21205, USA
* Corresponding author. Department of Veterans Affairs, Human Engineering Research Laboratories (HERL), VA Pittsburgh Healthcare System, 7180 Highland Drive, 151R-1, Pittsburgh, PA 15206.
E-mail address: dicianno@pitt.edu

Pediatr Clin N Am 57 (2010) 945–957
doi:10.1016/j.pcl.2010.07.014
0031-3955/10/$ – see front matter. Published by Elsevier Inc.

Spina bifida is a result of the incomplete development of the spinal cord and often results in paralysis, sensory deficits, and neurogenic bowel and bladder. Hydrocephalus is common and may result in cognitive impairments. Other neurologic issues such as Arnold Chiari Type II malformations, tethered cord syndrome, and syringomyelia may cause additional functional impairments. Additional issues may include orthopedic deformities, wounds, and renal complications. Management of the individual with spina bifida requires a comprehensive and multidisciplinary approach involving clinicians from many specialty areas such as physiatry, neurosurgery, neurology, urology, orthopedics, physical and occupational therapy, rehabilitation counseling, neuropsychology, and social services, as well as intensive nursing care.[1] Collaboration of care between these specialty areas provides a comprehensive and interdisciplinary approach to care for the child and family. Multidisciplinary collaboration may extend beyond the clinic or hospital setting as a child grows, enters school, expands his social circles, and transitions into his community as a teen or adult. Additional collaborative services at key transitional points in the child's development may involve school, vocational rehabilitation, and community outreach agencies.

In children with complex conditions like spina bifida, the usual developmental milestones may not be realized without specific attention and support. However, the multiple and medically demanding issues associated with spina bifida may preclude the necessary and time-sensitive assessment of developmental milestone achievement. A Life Course Model for patients, families, caregivers, teachers, and clinicians was developed with support by the National Spina Bifida Program, National Center on Birth Defects and Developmental Disabilities, Centers for Disease Control and Prevention, to facilitate a developmental approach to assessment and intervention along this life trajectory. This Life Course Model was then molded into a web-based tool that provides information about key developmental milestones for particular age groups, validated assessments that can be performed by clinicians or teachers to determine if milestones have been reached, useful suggestions for intervening in creative ways at each step, and evidence-based references. The Life Course Model is described in more detail in an accompanying by Mark Swanson article in this issue. However, a key concept is that the model describes life roles and milestones for the individual in childhood, school age, teen years, and adulthood. This model prepares the person for adult participation in roles related to the following domains: (1) self-management/health, (2) personal and social relationships, and (3) education/employment support. In creating the Life Course Model, clinicians and researchers from across the United States took a "reverse engineering" approach in identifying the developmental milestones one would need to master to successfully transition to adulthood.

In this article, the authors introduce the viewpoints of several key clinicians who are involved in the care of individuals with spina bifida and how the Life Course Model can assist them in the process of assessment, intervention, collaboration with other clinicians, and follow-up. A case study is used to demonstrate the experience of comprehensive and collaborative management in transitioning a child and his family from infancy to adulthood. This Life Course Model will be useful for all clinicians involved in the care of people with spina bifida, but may be a particularly valuable tool for any clinician who works outside a multidisciplinary setting or who may care for people with spina bifida on an infrequent basis.

In the Life Course Model the milestones, assessments, and interventions are different in each age period. Over the life span, the clinicians taking the more active roles in the transition process may change. In many clinics a nurse acts as a case manager, coordinating care among the various disciplines. In other instances a clinician may find that he or she must assist the individual and family even if care coordination is not his or her primary role. Regardless of who may be involved, the care coordination should always include emphasis on teamwork, loose boundaries around clinical roles, interventions that focus on promoting independence and preserving function, and support for caregivers.[2]

PHYSICIAN

The Life Course Model provides physicians with assessment tools that may help determine if patients are meeting age-appropriate developmental milestones in various areas. The model also provides many innovative, low-cost strategies not only in the treatment of many medical conditions common in spina bifida, but also for creative ways to educate patients and caregivers and to enhance compliance with self-care regimens. The model can be useful not only for the physician in the community who may lack the resources of large, multidisciplinary settings but also for the physician who is well versed in the care of those with spina bifida.

Many of the common diagnoses resulting in hospitalization and death in individuals with spina bifida are potentially preventable conditions.[3] Using the Life Course Model at each visit may help a physician to identify specific target areas where preventative care can be improved and to assess whether interventions provided at the last visit have made an objective or measurable difference. Physicians can also use the model during transitional visits, in which a young person is transitioning from a pediatric clinic either to an adult clinic or into the adult health care arena, because the model provides information on many of the medical and personal issues faced by a young person with spina bifida.

While there are many types of physicians who treat individuals with spina bifida, including those in primary care, pediatrics, and medical specialties, the care of the individual with spina bifida often requires teamwork among many providers. The Life Course Model can be used not only to foster collaborations between physicians and other clinicians such as therapists, neuropsychologists, nurses, or rehabilitation counselors, it can also prompt physicians as to when to consult a physician colleague. The ultimate goal of the model is to restore and preserve health and independent functioning using a team-based approach.

Breaches in skin integrity are one of the most important medical problems that can cause significant morbidity and mortality.[3] The Life Course Model provides physicians with tips on treating and preventing wounds, and education materials for patients and families on skin care. Tools are provided that may help the physician address some of the many causes of skin breakdown including nutritional status, pressure, shear, and moisture. Prompts are provided to remind physicians to evaluate for sensory deficits and how they may pose a threat to skin health.

Successful management of other issues such as neurogenic bowel and bladder also requires that the patient and caregivers work as a team with physicians. Besides medical or surgical interventions to manage incontinence and constipation, the physician plays a key role as an educator. The Life Course Model provides tools that may help the patient understand the importance of a bowel or bladder program, and gives tips on strategies for improving compliance and promoting continence.

Secondary musculoskeletal and neurologic disorders can have a significant impact on mobility. Some specialists such as physiatrists, neurosurgeons, developmental pediatricians, or orthopedists may routinely assess functional mobility and its relationship to developmental milestones at each visit. The Life Course Model, however, can guide other physicians in determining whether patients are meeting milestones, and provide suggestions on when referrals to other physician specialists or therapists are necessary, or when an assessment by a team of clinicians experienced in the prescription of orthoses or assistive technology is needed.

The Life Course Model also provides physicians with tools to promote health and wellness and to treat or prevent obesity, which has become a significant health concern.[4] Because not all individuals have access to nutritional support services, the physician may be one of the few sources of required information on diet and adaptive exercise. The model provides fun and creative suggestions for home exercise plans, dieting, and sports participation while taking into account such barriers as cost, transportation, motivation, or physical inaccessibility that many individuals face.

Physicians can also be a source of information for educational goals and gainful employment. The model provides physicians with information on when and how to make a referral for Vocational Rehabilitation, career counseling, or job shadowing services. Referrals to Vocational Rehabilitation programs may be necessary to secure funding for assistive technologies such as computer access devices, mobility equipment like wheelchairs, or adaptive driving evaluations and vehicle modifications. When educational or employment barriers are identified with help from the Life Course Model, the physician can offer guidance on which reasonable accommodations may be required. Of course, because a major barrier for education and employment is incontinence, managing the bowel and bladder can make a significant impact on outcomes in these areas. Physicians can also act as sounding boards for parents to develop realistic and medically appropriate goals for children and their teachers. This process may involve providing referrals to physical or occupational therapy or speech language pathology, Early Intervention (EI) services, or advocacy organizations including the Spina Bifida Association and its local chapters. The model provides suggestions for when this may be appropriate.

Given the high rate of acceptance of technology in this population,[5] physicians may also want to consider taking advantage of alternative technologies that may be available such as web-based or telerehabilitation systems. The model encourages the use of technology as a way to communicate and establish relationships with patients and other providers.

The physician can be involved in helping individuals with spina bifida and their families develop personal and social relationships in a healthy and age-appropriate way. The physician's role may involve identifying stressful issues within the family and support system, diagnosing anxiety or depression, screening for social skills at specific ages, and making referrals to teen clinics. Rarely do individuals with spina bifida obtain sexual education from physicians.[6] Most young adults desire more information on both fertility and sexuality.[7] The Life Course Model provides physicians with ways to assess and discuss sexuality and fertility for individuals of all ages.

Physicians wear the hats of educators and clinicians, but their roles as researchers also cannot be understated. Although much is known about the medical and rehabilitation management of spina bifida,[1] guidelines for evidence-based practice in many areas are still lacking, particularly in young adults. The Life Course Model can guide the academician in identifying those areas where research could advance the field substantially.

NURSE

Often in an advanced practice nursing role, the nurse has long been identified as instrumental for the patient and family in the transition process.[8] The coordinator's role is multifaceted[9] and the following roles may be needed: (1) expert nurse and coordinator of multidiscipline management, (2) patient and family advocate, (3) resource consultant, and (4) researcher. As the role of the spina bifida coordinator may vary in different multidisciplinary teams depending on educational background, job description, additional work responsibilities, team members, and size of clinic, the components of the nurse coordinator's clinical role in working with individuals with spina bifida and their families are now described.

The expert nurse and coordinator often works closely with the medical director of the spina bifida multidisciplinary team in managing the care of the patients during and between team visits. Using the nursing process of assessment, planning, implementing, and evaluating,[10] a plan of care is established with specialized medical professionals and allied health professionals at each visit. Recommendations made during a visit must be summarized and an ongoing plan of care established. This plan of care is vital to growth and development as the individual with spina bifida transitions from childhood to adulthood, expanding to his or her full potential. Between follow-up visits the plan of care may require diagnostic tests, referrals to physician specialists or therapists, follow-ups with primary care, or consults with a dietician, neuropsychologist, or social worker. The nurse coordinator is many times the professional responsible for consolidating a written or verbal report from all multidiscipline specialties evaluating the individual with spina bifida in a clinical setting, making sure the individual and family has a copy of the recommendations, and discussing and clarifying direction for the individual with spina bifida and their family between visits. The nurse coordinator works as a liaison to link the various personnel involved in the care plan and those in community outreach to assist the individual and family in obtaining the care recommended by the multidisciplinary team. The nurse coordinator assists with communication to the various care providers, providing clarification, modification, and feedback among professionals.

The expert nurse and coordinator also acts as a first-line professional in triage when an individual with spina bifida or caregiver calls with a concern or problem between clinic visits. The nurse, as a clinician with expertise and knowledge about spina bifida, may be able to resolve many triage concerns. Unexpected crises and unplanned events can easily result in delays and regression in meeting transitional goals. The nurse coordinator, as a clinician, provides prompt follow-up and response from the spina bifida multidisciplinary team and assists in redirecting the individual and family with spina bifida back to the transitional goals established, or initiates modification of those goals if needed. The Life Course Model can be valuable in allowing the nurse coordinator to follow and assess a patient's developmental milestones, and allowing intervention by rapidly triaging problems and activating needed interventions and consultations. The nurse coordinator and other team members can use the Life Course Model to ensure all team members are working toward the patient's and caregivers' necessary and agreed-upon goals.

People with spina bifida and their caregivers may lack information about self-advocacy. The expert nurse and coordinator, acting as an advocate, can provide this education. For example, parents often need to learn to work with their child's school to ensure access to all services that are deemed necessary for the child to thrive and succeed in school. This collaboration may include learning needs of the child, finding a private place for the child to catheterize, or finding access to adaptive playground equipment or an elevator for a child who uses a wheelchair. The nurse provides leadership and support in this process. The nurse often takes the lead in teaching individuals and families that cognitive impairments and learning disabilities can interfere with the development and accomplishment of personal care skills and functional independence.[11] The Life Course Model provides not only the nurse coordinator but also the patient and families with valuable tools and suggestions for advocacy and understanding patients' rights.

Nurses act as resource consultants because they are on the front line of care in the lives of individuals with spina bifida and their families.[11] Nurses keep a current knowledge of resources that are available for individuals with spina bifida. Informational Web resources such as the Spina Bifida Association of America (SBAA), or state, regional, and community resources are identified and offered to families on a wide variety of topics. If information is not known, the nurse is often able to investigate and find resources. Coordinating follow-up care involves making parents aware of resources and support networks for families on the local, regional, and national level.[9] The Life Course Model provides the nurse with an extensive list of ideas and resources.

Nurses are also scientists and play the role of researchers. Because nurses are intimately involved in the lives of their patients and families, they are well suited to identifying areas of necessary research, promoting academic work that is clinically relevant, and translating research findings into evidence-based practice. The Life Course Model can serve as a research tool to allow clinician-researchers to identify key research priorities.

OCCUPATIONAL THERAPIST

Occupational therapists (OTs) view the person, the environment, and the interaction between persons and their environments in a holistic manner. Persons continually adapt to the environments in which they live, work, and play while influencing the environment. There is a dynamic interaction created through the individual's life-long learning, development, and maturation. Likewise, the environment is also continually evolving and changing, at times in response to the individual's needs and actions as well as in response to external variables. The developmental frame of reference was originally identified by Lela Llorens, an occupational therapist. The model is built on social, psychological, and physical aspects of life tasks and relationships.[12] Llorens[13] focused on 2 perspectives: (1) the specific period of life (horizontal development) and (2) the course of time (longitudinal development). The Life Course Model is similarly structured according to developmental milestones that we strive to achieve at various phases of life.

OTs work with persons who have spina bifida in a variety of settings. El services for children from birth to age 3 years typically occur in the home or daycare setting. Developmentally, this is a period in our lives in which the greatest amount of change occurs in the shortest amount of time. OTs working in El may not be considering what skills will make their patient a successful employee or spouse, but often focus on assisting them in achieving more immediate developmental milestones. When developmental delay is present and certain skills are not readily emerging, it can eventually cause an incongruity, with some areas of development being advanced and others lagging. Once we reach later stages of development these incongruities become more apparent as several skill areas are often required to complete activities and fulfill more complex roles. Furthermore, an El OT may only have 1 or 2 patients on their caseload with a diagnosis of spina bifida. Although the El OT may be experienced and skilled at his or her profession as a clinician, the diversity of diagnoses in patient caseload is broad and time is further limited by travel to the various locations where patients are seen for treatment. The Life Course Model helps to ensure that no areas are overlooked and that assessments and interventions are readily available for the therapist's and family's access.

This tool continues to assist OTs who work in school-based settings. School-based OTs treat students from ages 3 to 21 years. Again, pediatric OTs who work in public or private settings may have just 1 or 2 students registered for treatment on their caseloads. The process for identifying needs and ongoing goals in the school setting occurs through the development and updates of the students' Individual Education Plan (IEP). Despite having only 1 or 2 students on a caseload who have spina bifida, rehabilitation professionals working in school settings tend to have more experience than other members of the IEP team, including teachers and social workers. Use of the Life Course Model as part of the IEP process helps to ensure that no areas of intervention that can be implemented to further support and enhance the skills of the student are overlooked. Beginning at age 14 years, students in the IEP process should be integrating goals and objectives that prepare the student for transition following high school graduation, whether this includes postsecondary education, employment, or other activities relevant for successful participation as an adult. This is a critical time for the young person to be participating in opportunities that will enable him or her to transition to successful adult roles and include planning for postsecondary education, employment, and independent living.

Once a person with spina bifida has reached adulthood, the most common treatment settings include acute inpatient, skilled nursing facilities, or home health. Often the duration of OT treatment as adult is typically much briefer than in earlier years. However, the Life Course Model is still relevant, and the resources provided can be an invaluable source of information for busy clinicians as they assist in discharge planning, develop home programs, and participate in the education of persons with spina bifida and caregivers.

Finally, OTs are also often members of the team of professionals who work at both pediatric and adult spina bifida clinics. This setting is perhaps that in which the model can best be implemented because of the long-term (often life-long) nature of treatment by a team of professionals dedicated to the care, rehabilitation, and support of persons with spina bifida.

REHABILITATION COUNSELOR

Regardless of the role that the rehabilitation counselor plays in service provision, having a single resource to provide developmental milestones, as well as the means of assessing and addressing progress toward these milestones, will serve to improve the quality and specialization of the services provided, especially because many rehabilitation counselors do not have a specialized knowledge of spina bifida.

Rehabilitation counselors perform 4 primary functions when working with individuals with spina bifida and their families. When working with individuals with spina bifida, rehabilitation counselors act as counselors and case managers. When working with families of or organizations providing services to individuals with spina bifida, rehabilitation counselors serve as consultants and advocates.[14] More specifically, depending on the setting in which the rehabilitation counselor provides services, tasks may include diagnosis, assessment, development planning and follow-through, placement and follow-up services, postemployment services, and general service provision.[15] The comprehensive Life Course Model proposed here provides a resource framework across the life span that can be used by rehabilitation counselors, particularly given their multifaceted roles and the variety of settings across which they might work.

When the rehabilitation counselor acts as a counselor, he or she provides therapeutic and psychoeducational services; this can include working with individuals, groups, or families.[14] In this regard, the Life Course Model provides information for understanding and assessing the relationships and social interactions of individuals with spina bifida. In addition, information regarding the developmental milestones and the degree to which they have been met, as well as the information on assessment and intervention for these milestones provided by the Life Course Model, will assist in the development of appropriate goals and goal planning.

The rehabilitation counselor also acts as a case manager, and may use the multidisciplinary components and developmental tracking provided by the Life Course Model. A case manager "organizes, coordinates, and sustains a network of formal and informal supports and activities designed to optimize the well-being and functioning of people with multiple needs."[14] The Life Course Model provides the organizational structure and basis for coordinating services, assessing needs, and communicating with individuals and their families. The division of needs assessment in the model into areas of health, relationships, and education/income support, along with associated landmarks and tools for assessment and intervention, provides a valuable tool for case management.

The rehabilitation counselor also acts as a consultant. In much the same way that the Life Course Model serves rehabilitation counselors in their role as case managers, it provides a framework and basis for communication in their role as consultants. Consultation may occur with individuals, families, groups, organizations, or communities, and may address communication, decision making, coping skills, remediation services, job-enrichment programs, or reducing the impact of functional disability.[14] Situations in which consultation occurs vary across the life span and across settings and service providers. The ability to communicate across these various settings and with individuals, families, and professionals using a common language and a common framework assists in streamlining the process of consultation and the move from consultation to action and intervention.

The best advocate knows the strengths, abilities, and needs of the individuals they serve. When the rehabilitation counselor is an advocate, his or her ultimate goal is to change "environments for growth and development."[14] The Life Course Model provides information about the individual's needs, strengths, abilities, and environments, and serves as a tool for growth and change.

Rehabilitation counselors most often work with individuals with spina bifida in vocational rehabilitation. The vocational barriers and needs of individuals with spina bifida span the health, social, and educational domains, and have been found to include bladder control, ambulation, pressure sores, poor job retention, lack of assistance in job searching and placement, poor health insurance, discrimination, lack of career preparation, and lack of involvement in planning the rehabilitation process.[16–18] The Life Course Model may best serve rehabilitation counselors in vocational rehabilitation by improving the intervention and prevention of many of these barriers earlier in the life span. It also provides rehabilitation counselors with the ability to track, assess, and recommend interventions with the ultimate goal of improving employment outcomes.

In all the roles assumed by rehabilitation counselors, the ability to gather information, communicate with individuals, families, and organizations using a common language, and the access to resources for assessment and intervention only serves to enhance service provision. The Life Course Model, therefore, will improve service provision and allow for more individualized and client-centered counseling, case management, consultation, and advocacy.

NEUROPSYCHOLOGIST

Neuropsychological assessment and consultation is a useful means of identifying the strengths or weaknesses of individuals with spina bifida, identifying intervention/accommodation needs, and monitoring the stability of mental status in this potentially unstable neurologic condition. Repeated neuropsychological assessment is often performed across the early life span of individuals with spina bifida, for several reasons. First, neuropsychological assessment can assist in the early identification of spina bifida–related learning difficulties that create distinct challenges for educational teams at different points in the educational process (eg, early delays demonstrated in preschool math abilities, reading comprehension difficulties displayed in later elementary school, organizational problems shown in middle school and high school). Second, neuropsychological assessment can be sensitive to the cognitive impact of hydrocephalus, both as a potential indicator of shunt failure and as a method of quantifying cognitive changes associated with past hydrocephalic episodes.[19] Third, neuropsychological assessment is useful for identifying cognitive, behavioral, and emotional variables that can interfere in the ability of individuals with spina bifida to meet increases in self-management expectations (eg, medical self-care, activities of daily living) as they occur across the early life span.[20]

The Life Course Model is a useful resource in each of these assessment scenarios, as it provides an additional developmental context for individuals with spina bifida at different stages of development. Under the first assessment scenario (assessment targeted toward identification of spina bifida–related learning difficulties), the information contained in the Life Course Model provides the assessing neuropsychologist with specific information regarding learning disability in spina bifida, frequently used tests to identify these disabilities, and a variety of suggested interventions culled from research literature, anecdotal reports, or clinician expertise. While neuropsychologists are trained in many of the cognitive and learning problems identified in youth with developmental disabilities, the Life Course Model resource provides additional information specific to spina bifida for assessment-related purposes.

Under the second assessment scenario (quantifying cognitive changes associated with hydrocephalic episodes), the Life Course Model provides information that would be helpful for interpreting reported symptoms, particularly those that might occur with considerable regularity in youth with spina bifida. For instance, considerable information is provided in the Life Course Model regarding initiation deficits that are often noted in youth with spina bifida. When youths with spina bifida are placed in new situations in which additional self-initiative is necessary, they can often appear to have "regressed" or "declined" in functioning because more problems are being reported than noted in similar situations in the past (eg, increased report of poor homework completion when the youth with spina bifida is promoted into high school where additional organizational skills and individual initiative are required). The developmental context provided by the Life Course Model provides additional information to help the neuropsychologist determine if a true change in functioning has occurred (suggestive of shunt failure), or if these "changes" can be linked to new environmental challenges instead.

The Life Course Model is useful for neuropsychologists testing youth with spina bifida under the third testing scenario (ie, identifying cognitive, behavioral, and emotional variables that can interfere in the ability to meet self-management expectations). Neuropsychologists are adept at quantifying cognitive strengths and weaknesses, including areas such as working memory, prospective memory, and organizational skills that may have considerable relevance to the self-management of a condition such as spina bifida. The Life Course Model provides the neuropsychologist with a comprehensive overview of the various self-management skills and self-care competencies that eventually become the responsibility of adolescents and young adults with spina bifida (eg, self-catheterization, obesity prevention, skin care). By providing neuropsychologists with this specialized information, the neuropsychologist can identify functional areas in which the youth may be at risk (eg, skin breakdown due to failure to initiate pressure relief exercises) given his or her specific areas of neuropsychological weakness, rather than simply identifying general areas of neurocognitive deficit (eg, poor initiation).

Finally, the Life Course Model provides the neuropsychologist with an interpersonal context in which to understand the youth with spina bifida. Areas such as friendship, parent/child interaction, relationship with siblings, and development of intimate/romantic relationships are all core components of social functioning and identity development. The specialized information available within the Life Course Model provides neuropsychologists with valuable information regarding how those around the youth can respond to his or her pattern of strengths or weaknesses, and help facilitate healthy interpersonal development.

LONGITUDINAL CASE STUDY
Birth to 3 Years

Julio has been participating in EI services based on his Individualized Family Service Plan (IFSP), and sees his OT weekly. His OT, based on the recommended assessment tools in the Life Course Model, administers the Wee-FIM and determines that Julio has deficits in early object usage. In addition, discussion with his family reveals that they have concerns about Julio's physical safety when opportunities arise for him to interact with nondisabled peers, which has limited any such interaction. After reviewing recommendations for possible interventions and determining what was most appropriate for Julio's situation, his OT discusses the importance of Julio engaging in parallel play activities within the community. He begins participating in a swim program appropriate for his age group and attended by young children and their parents. His OT also provides information to Julio's parents regarding developmentally appropriate toys that encourage understanding of cause and effect relationships. The nurse coordinator discusses these events with Julio's OT and refers Julio's parents to a local support group found via the Web site resources. Julio's parents then began interacting with other families who have children with spina bifida. His primary care physician provides anticipatory guidance, well child care, acute care for illness, immunizations, growth, and nutrition follow-up, as well as input into development of the IFSP.

Years 3 to 5

Julio has been attending a local Head Start program designed to accommodate children with developmental disabilities. Julio has been using a walker and often is unable to quickly engage in floor-time play with his peers due to difficulty in transferring from stand to sit position and clutter of the environment (eg, peers on the floor, toys). While working on ambulation goals with his physical therapist (PT), the PT consults the Life Course Model Web site. While thinking more about his ambulation goals, she finds ways to organize the play space differently to allow for clear walkways. Also, the Head Start program develops several play areas enabling Julio to interact with his peers in a standing position. At the next clinic visit, the nurse coordinator discusses Julio's mobility with his family, using a list of mobility milestones she obtained from the Web site. She communicates Julio's achievements and goals to the team of clinicians scheduled to see him. His primary care physician continues health supervision and anticipatory guidance, monitors growth and nutrition, provides immunizations, and communicates with the Early Childhood Special Education program (Part B), which works with the Head Start program to provide developmentally appropriate intervention services, based on Julio's IEP.

School Years

Up until the fourth grade, Julio has been successful academically. However, his math teacher has noticed he is now struggling to keep up with the rest of the students. His IEP does not specifically address any type of learning disability. Julio's parents, on receiving notice from his math teacher about his struggles, access the Life Course Model Web site and recognize that this is a milestone their son may not yet have achieved. Concerned, they complete the Nonverbal Learning Disabilities (NLD), a Parent Rating Scale recommended by the Web site. Based on the results from this scale, his parents request further evaluation by a neuropsychologist to determine if Julio has an NLD. Based on the results from this assessment, Julio's IEP is adapted to reflect the new information. Julio's parents also provide feedback to Julio's teachers based on what they learned from the Web site. His primary care physician continues to provide health supervision, anticipatory guidance, and monitors the IEP.

Teen

Julio is now 15 years old and has been in high school. The school administers a typical interest inventory for students to begin thinking about future careers. Julio's guidance/rehabilitation counselor is concerned, as Julio still expresses a desire only to pursue a career as a professional rap star. He is unwilling to consider other options and believes that his goal is realistic. Julio's counselor consults the Life Course Model Web site for further inventories to assess Julio's strengths and abilities. She chooses the Work-Adjustment Inventory to assess Julio's work temperament and the Jacobs Pre-Vocational Assessment (JPVA) to asses his specific work-related skills. Based on the results from these assessments, Julio's counselor helps him find a volunteer opportunity in the community in line with his interests and abilities. In addition, she encourages Julio to explore rapping as a hobby and to perform in a local or school variety show. His counselor also sets up a peer mentor through the local SBAA chapter and encourages Julio's parents to provide him with opportunities to interact with other adults to discuss potential career paths. His primary care physician continues to provide health care supervision on adolescent issues such as sexuality, risky behavior, and substance abuse, as well as monitoring the transition plan of the IEP.

Adult

Julio has recently moved into his own apartment and uses public transportation to get around the community. He has been using a manual wheelchair for mobility. He has a part-time job at a local department store and plays wheelchair basketball with the local men's team. Julio's employer contacts his rehabilitation counselor with concerns over recent complaints from coworkers regarding Julio's personal hygiene. The rehabilitation counselor meets with Julio to discuss the problem. Julio is adamant that he has not been experiencing incontinence on the job, and that he washes his clothes and showers before going to work. Although she believes that Julio is telling the truth, the counselor also notices a strong odor. She accesses the Life Course Model Web site and learns that skin breakdown can be a significant issue for those with spina bifida and can cause strong odor as well. She also recognizes that Julio should be making regular appointments with health care providers specializing in maintaining his health status. She refers him to the nearest adult spina bifida clinic. The nurse coordinator speaks with Julio, and gives him additional information on skin care and pressure relief maneuvers that she found through links in the Life Course Model Web site. She sets him up to see a physiatrist in the clinic to treat the pressure ulcer and obtain a new cushion. The physiatrist previously found a PT who specializes in seating assessments by consulting professional organizations listed in the Life Course Model Web site. The physiatrist and PT work as a team to prescribe a new cushion and refer him back to his rehabilitation counselor to discuss funding options for the new equipment through the vocational rehabilitation program. Julio's rehabilitation counselor sets up a meeting with Julio's employer to explain the situation regarding his health. She helps him to fill out any necessary paperwork and they request a medical leave of absence until Julio is able to return to work again. In addition, she helps Julio to set up reminders to perform daily skin checks. Together they consult the Web site for ideas. She and Julio decide that a laminated reminder in his shower and a daily alarm on his Smart Phone to confirm that he has completed his skin check should help prevent this from occurring in the future.

SUMMARY

The care of a person with spina bifida requires multidisciplinary care from a variety of health care professionals. As a child grows and develops, the circle of providers enlarges to include community as well as new support systems and health care providers. Collaboration of all of these services and providers is important to the development and transition to adulthood for the child and family. The Life Course Model can be used by the patients, their families, and those clinicians involved in the growing child's care to assist in development of the individual with spina bifida to live as independently and successfully as possible.

REFERENCES

1. Dicianno BE, Kurowski BG, Yang JMJ, et al. Rehabilitation and medical management of the adult with spina bifida. Am J Phys Med Rehabil 2008;87(12):1027.
2. Rapport MK, McWilliams RA, Smith BJ. Practices across disciplines in early intervention. Infants Young Child 2004;17(1):32–44.
3. Dicianno BE, Wilson RW. Hospitalizations of adults with spina bifida and congenital spinal cord anomalies. Arch Phys Med Rehabil 2010;91(4):529–35.
4. Dosa NP, Foley JT, Eckrich M, et al. Obesity across the lifespan among persons with spina bifida. Disabil Rehabil 2009;31(11):914–20.
5. Dicianno BE, Gaines A, Collins DM, et al. Mobility, assistive technology use, and social integration among adults with spina bifida. Am J Phys Med Rehabil 2009; 88(7):533.
6. Cardenas DD, Topolski TD, White CJ, et al. Sexual functioning in adolescents and young adults with spina bifida. Arch Phys Med Rehabil 2008;89(1):31–5.
7. Sawyer SM, Roberts KV. Sexual and reproductive health in young people with spina bifida. Dev Med Child Neurol 1999;41(10):671–5.
8. Peterson P, Rauen K, Brown J, et al. Spina bifida: the transition into adulthood begins in infancy. Rehabil Nurs 1994;19:220–38.
9. Dunleavy MJ. The role of the nurse coordinator in spina bifida clinics. Scientific World Journal 2007;26(7):1884–9.
10. Jarvis C. Physical examination and health assessment. Canada: Saunders; 2008. p. 2–4.
11. Braun P, Brown J. Care of the child with altered neurophysiological function. In: Votroubek W, Tabacco A, editors. Pediatric home care for nurses: a family centered approach. 1st edition. Boston (MA): Jones and Bartlett; 2009. p. 107–8, Chapter 6.
12. Llorens LA. Facilitating growth and development: the promise of occupational therapy. Am J Occup Ther 1969;24:93–101.

13. Llorens LA. Application of developmental theory for health and rehabilitation. Rockville (MD): American Occupational Therapy Association; 1976.
14. Riggar TF, Maki DR. Concepts and paradigms, handbook of rehabilitation counseling. New York: Springer Publishing Company; 2004. p. 1–24.
15. Rubin SE, Roessler RT. The role and function of the rehabilitation counselor, foundations of the vocational rehabilitation process. 5th edition. Austin (TX): Pro-ed; 2001. p. 257–66.
16. Singh U, Gogia VS. Rehabilitation of patients with spina bifida. Indian J Pediatr 1997;64(6):77–82.
17. Lonton AP, Loughlin AM, Dunleavy M. The role of the nurse coordinator in spina bifida clinics. Scientific World Journal 2007;7:1884–9.
18. Schreiner K, Roessler R, Johnson P. Identifying employment concerns of people with spina bifida. J Appl Rehabil Counsel 1993;24(2):22–37.
19. Matson M, Mahone EM, Zabel TA. Serial neuropsychological assessment and evidence of shunt malfunction in spina bifida: a longitudinal case study. Child Neuropsychol 2005;11(4):315–32.
20. Tarazi R, Mahone EM, Zabel TA. Self-care independence in children with neurological disorders: an interactional model of adaptive demands and executive dysfunction. Rehabil Psychol 2007;52(2):196–205.

Implementing a Specialty Electronic Medical Record to Document a Life-Course Developmental Model and Facilitate Clinical Interventions in Spina Bifida Clinics

Andrea D. Fairman, MOT, OTR/L, CPRP[a,*], Judy K. Thibadeau, RN, MN[b],
Brad E. Dicianno, MD[c,d], Bambang Parmanto, PhD[e]

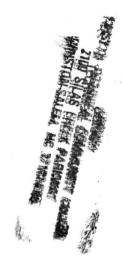

KEYWORDS

- Electronic medical record • Spina bifida
- Developmental model • Transition

Statement of financial support: This work was supported by the National Spina Bifida Program, National Center on Birth Defects and Developmental Disabilities, Centers for Disease Control and Prevention, Atlanta, Georgia.

The authors have nothing to disclose. The findings and conclusions in this report are those of the authors and do not necessarily represent the official position of the Centers for Disease Control and Prevention.

[a] Department of Rehabilitation Science and Technology, University of Pittsburgh, School of Health and Rehabilitation Sciences, Forbes Tower, Suite 5044, 3600 Forbes Avenue, Pittsburgh, PA 15260, USA

[b] Division of Human Development and Disability, National Center on Birth Defects and Developmental Disabilities, Centers for Disease Control and Prevention, 1600 Clifton Road, Mailstop E-88, Atlanta, GA 30033, USA

[c] Department of Veterans Affairs, Human Engineering Research Laboratories (HERL), VA Pittsburgh Healthcare System, 7180 Highland Drive, 151R-1, Pittsburgh, PA 15206, USA

[d] Department of Physical Medicine and Rehabilitation, University of Pittsburgh Medical Center (UPMC), Kaufmann Medical Building, Suite 202, 3471 5th Avenue, Pittsburgh, PA 15213, USA

[e] Department of Health Information Management, University of Pittsburgh School of Health and Rehabilitation Sciences, 6026 Forbes Tower, 3600 Forbes Avenue, Pittsburgh, PA 15260, USA

* Corresponding author.
E-mail address: adf29@pitt.edu

Pediatr Clin N Am 57 (2010) 959–971
doi:10.1016/j.pcl.2010.07.015
0031-3955/10/$ – see front matter © 2010 Elsevier Inc. All rights reserved.

pediatric.theclinics.com

Many young adults with disabilities are reaching adulthood without the skills to successfully use the adult health system or to support themselves.[1] Children with disabilities move through the usual childhood development stages as do their nondisabled peers, yet they face additional challenges that accompany their specific condition.[2] When the issues of self-care, education, employment, and independent living are not addressed early in life, lack of attention to these issues may negatively impact the future achievement of developmental milestones. The young person may struggle in caring for him or herself and may not make the transition to adult living with the associated health care choices.[3]

Advances in medical technology have increased the life expectancy of children born with spina bifida (SB).[4–6] Until the last several decades, these children were not expected to live to adulthood; thus, plans for life after childhood were not made or considered. In a study of all live infants born with SB between 1979 to 1994 in Atlanta, Georgia, the survival rate to 1 year was 87.2%, and to 18 years, 78.4%.[7] This is the first generation where larger numbers of persons with SB are surviving to reach adulthood. However, little is known regarding best practices to aide young persons with SB in achieving successful transition to adult roles such as: employment, independent living, and effective self-management of health routines. The "Evidence-Based Practice in Spina Bifida" conference was convened in Washington, DC, in 2003 to identify research and practice priorities. The dearth of sound research on which current treatments are based was detailed by Liptak[8] in the conference proceedings. Evidence-based research is lacking regarding the multiple and complex issues that affect medical, social, and psychological aspects of life for children with SB, which may impede their transition to independence as adults.

Over the past several years, the Spina Bifida Association (SBA) and the Centers for Disease Control and Prevention (CDC) have collaborated to develop the National Spina Bifida Program in an effort to address the need for increased research in SB. A life course model to facilitate a developmental approach to realize healthy, satisfying participation in adult life has been developed for persons affected by SB.[9] Children with complex conditions like SB, may not reach the usual developmental milestones without specific attention and support. The multiple and medically demanding issues associated with conditions like SB may preclude the necessary and time sensitive assessment of developmental milestone achievement.

Mechanisms to allow for pooling of data across SB clinics throughout the United States include the development of a patient registry and the SB electronic medical record (EMR). As described below, the purpose of the SB EMR is to improve clinical care by promoting the systematic collection of demographic, intervention, and outcome data. Those clinics participating in the initial version of the patient registry have the opportunity to use the SB EMR to collect patient registry and other clinical data. Additional information regarding the patient registry is discussed later in this article. The SB EMR will eventually integrate the developmental life-course model to include age-specific prompts facilitating the clinician's and family's identification of the individual's achievement of developmental milestones. If milestones are not being accomplished within the appropriate age-range, the current Life-Course Model web site can also provide the measure of milestone accomplishment, recommendations of interventions to assist with the milestone, and the follow-up that may provide attention to this important part of growing up to achieve self-sufficiency as an adult.

THE NATIONAL SPINA BIFIDA PROGRAM

To enhance the knowledge regarding care effectiveness, a national SB clinic survey was conducted in 2005, by the Delmarva Foundation, to explore clinic staffing, patient load, funding, strengths, perceived needs, and involvement in clinical research and quality improvement activities.[10] The survey respondents included professionals of varying disciplines knowledgeable about the functioning of the clinics (ie, nurses, physicians, therapists). The conclusions drawn, based on an analysis of the survey by the Delmarva Foundation, are:

- Great variability exists in care across clinics and greater standardization of care is needed. There is a need for clearer agreement regarding the set of services that should be available in all SB clinics and prospective patients and their families should be able to know which services and staff they can expect at any SB clinic in the country.
- Clinics need better coordination and sharing of information in order to support research and quality improvement activities. Although many clinics are involved in research and quality improvement initiatives, no mechanism exists for pooling data across clinics to better understand how care can be improved. A coordinated effort is needed to collect key data about clinics' financing and organization and the services they provide to be able to link those to patient outcomes. Such data can help to identify areas where improvements in quality are needed as well as where research needs to be conducted. Information across clinics will enable clinics to apply for cross-center funding and establish a greater evidence base for care in SB.

The conclusions of this survey prompted the SBA Professional Advisory Council to recommend the development of a national infrastructure to support clinical research and a systematic approach to improving quality of care. This was translated into the need for a network of SB clinics and for a SB patient registry in order that there could be a national perspective regarding the structure and care delivered in SB clinics.

WEB-BASED SB EMR

To reduce the variability of care delivered in SB clinics nationally, to identify SB care improvement opportunities, and to build a platform of future research for this very rare condition, the SBA, in collaboration with the CDC and local partners, embarked on a process to build a network of SB clinics and a registry of patients who receive care in those clinics. In order for the registry data to be collected via a standardized, electronic process before transfer to the designated repository, the program worked with a software vendor to develop a web-based SB EMR. An EMR is intended to automatically store each symptom, sign, result, and assessment for every patient. Common advantages of EMRs are decrease in cost and improvement in quality of care through reduction of medical errors.[11] An EMR is described by Aspden and colleagues[12] in the *2003 Institute of Medicine Patient Safety Report* as encompassing:

- A longitudinal collection of electronic health information for and about persons
- Immediate electronic access to person- and population-level information by authorized users
- Provision of knowledge and decision-support systems that enhance the quality, safety, and efficiency of patient care
- Support for efficient processes for health care delivery.

EMRs have been proposed and proven as a sustainable solution for improving the quality of medical care.[13] A sample of the functionality offered in the SB EMR is as follows:

- The ability to track patient demographics (**Fig. 1**), educational interventions (**Fig. 2**), providers, consents, visits (**Fig. 3**), insurance, laboratory results,

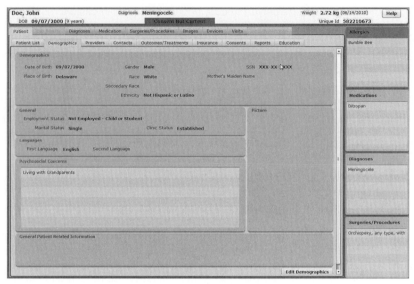

Fig. 1. SB EMR. Screen shot: patient demographics.

medications, allergies, diagnoses, infections, surgeries or procedures, assistive devices (**Fig. 4**), and information on gait, mobility and continence
- Pick lists, providing choice of selected terms in a window, that default to SB-specific content for convenient data entry
- A display of laboratory results in spreadsheet format entry and view of medications by either brand or generic names
- Note fields containing a lock mechanism to ensure that data are protected from accidental revision or deletion.

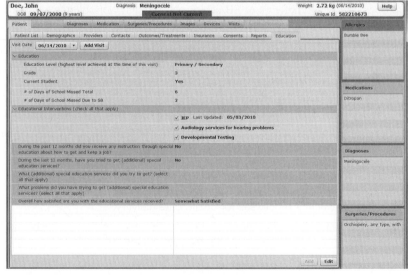

Fig. 2. SB EMR. Screen shot: educational interventions.

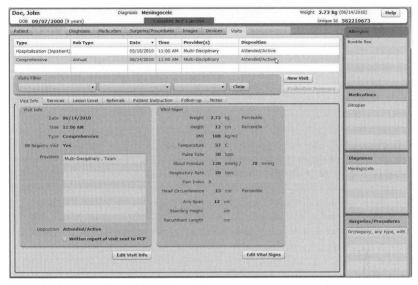

Fig. 3. SB EMR. Screen shot: visits information.

This application has been developed to comply with current and future National Institute of Standards Technology.[14] The following internationally recognized, standardized vocabularies and databases have also been included in the development of the SB EMR to enhance the capacity of data mining and sharing.

Systemized Nomenclature of Medicine Clinical Terms (SNOMED CT) is a dynamic, scientifically validated, clinical health care terminology and infrastructure that makes health care information more usable and accessible. The SNOMED CT core

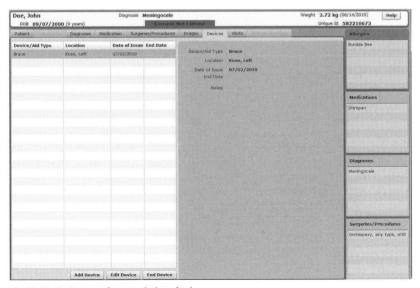

Fig. 4. SB EMR. Screen shot: assistive devices.

terminology provides a common language that enables a consistent way of capturing, sharing, and aggregating health data across specialties and sites of care. Software suppliers, government entities, and health care organizations in over 30 countries have adopted SNOMED CT since its release in January, 2002. National government agreements include the United Kingdom National Health Service, the Australian Health Service, and the United States National Library of Medicine.[15] The SB EMR Development Committee selected SNOMED CT to serve as the foundation for the application's structured vocabulary. This will help to ensure the long-term interoperability of the application and enhance the ability to contribute data to national and international clinical research and surveillance.

Logical Observation Identifiers Names and Codes (LOINC) is a database for identifying medical laboratory observations. LOINC was created in response to the demand for an electronic database for clinical care and management. LOINC applies universal code names and identifiers to medical terminology related to the electronic health record. The purpose is to assist in the electronic exchange and gathering of clinical results (such as laboratory tests, clinical observations, outcomes management, and research).[16]

First Databank's National Drug Data File Plus (NDDF Plus) is the industry's most widely used drug database. NDDF Plus combines comprehensive drug attributes and pricing information with an extensive array of clinical decision-support modules. It encompasses medications approved by the FDA, plus information on alternative-therapy agents such as herbals, nutraceuticals, and dietary supplements.[17]

The International Statistical Classification of Diseases and Related Health Problems (ICD) provides codes to classify diseases and a wide variety of signs, symptoms, abnormal findings, complaints, social circumstances, and external causes of injury or disease. Under this system, every health condition can be assigned to a unique category and given a code, up to six characters long. Such categories can include a set of similar diseases. The ICD is published by the World Health Organization (WHO) and used worldwide for morbidity and mortality statistics, reimbursement systems, and automated decision support in medicine. This system is designed to promote international comparability in the collection, processing, classification, and presentation of these statistics. The ICD is a core classification of the WHO Family of International Classifications (WHO-FIC). The US National Library of Medicine (NLM) has released a draft of rules-based mapping from SNOMED CT to the ICD, 9th revision, Clinical Modification (ICD-9-CM).[18] The map was designed to support semiautomated administrative reporting and reimbursement for health care services within United States health care organizations. The use of both SNOMED CT and the ICD-9-CM coding system is a possibility in the near future and will be included in the SB EMR. Use of these standardized systems and terminology will help to ensure the consistency in collection and pooling of data within the SB EMR to study larger numbers of persons with respect to clinical outcomes.

Use of web-based EMRs for enhancing cross-institutional clinical care and research is not a new concept.[19] The hemophilia and cystic fibrosis communities have collected clinic specific information for several decades using standard data collection formats that have evolved over time and have been used as models in developing the SB EMR. The Hemophilia Treatment Center (HTC) model of care is multidisciplinary and integrates intensive patient and family education in its core philosophy. The HTC model demonstrates "how successful partnerships among health care professionals, consumers, and government agencies have created a nationwide regional health delivery system that has optimized access to care and prevention services and improved health outcomes for people with hemophilia in the United States."[20] Likewise, the Cystic Fibrosis Foundation has demonstrated the value of a registry and importance of guidelines for patient care. Systematically, the cystic fibrosis registry collects and documents valuable information regarding natural history and evaluates the effectiveness of new interventions using factor analysis.[21] The experiences of these two rare conditions were explored in depth as the plans for the SB network of clinics and the patient registry were proceeding. There have been multiple improvements in methods of service delivery and outcomes of care for persons with cystic fibrosis and persons with hemophilia as a result of these efforts.[20,21]

EMR USAGE OF UNITED STATES SPINA BIFIDA CLINICS—A BRIEF SURVEY

Typically, SB clinics exist within the context of larger health care systems, such as private hospitals and university affiliated institutions. Many of these health care systems' EMRs provide a generic approach to the collection of patient data and are not customized to gather clinical data specific to the SB population. As a result, information that is relevant and specific to the care of persons with SB may not be adequately captured in the EMR. There has been little progress made on the adoption of a universal, national EMR.[22]

A brief survey of the SB clinics in the United States was conducted through the SBA's professional listserv in March, 2010. This inquiry was intended to gain an understanding of the clinics' current usage of EMRs to collect and track clinical data. Questions were also posed regarding the possible barriers to the adoption of the web-based SB EMR. Although only 16 clinics, representing a small portion of the 162 clinics in the United States, responded to the survey, together these 16 clinics provide care to approximately 6,000 persons with spina bifida. Of the 16 clinics that responded, 13 (81%) already have one or more EMR systems in place.

The 13 clinics that use EMRs indicated use of six distinct EMR software programs. One of the institutions has developed their own unique EMR system that is not commercially available. **Table 1** lists five commercially available EMRs and functionalities (note that new functionalities are always being added to EMR software; this list represents vendor-released specifications at the time this article was written but may not be fully comprehensive). Although some EMRs being used are quite comprehensive, several shortcomings common to all five make them inadequate for the type of charting needed in the SB population. First, even if a single data system were in use at all institutions, data may not be shared universally across institutions. Although clinicians within a network of hospitals at a university, for example, can view a patient's chart, if the patient sees a clinician in a different network using the same EMR system, the patient's chart likely will not be accessible at the other site. Second, some EMRs being used were originally developed as inpatient EMRs and were later modified for the outpatient setting. This limits the ability of the system to provide charting capabilities that mimic the typical workflow of a clinic. As a result, many centers use one EMR for inpatients and one for outpatients, and there may be problems with data sharing between those systems. Finally, although some specifications list that EMR systems are technically supposed to interface with other accessibility software for users with disabilities, such as voice recognition or screen reading software, the performance may not be seamless.

An interesting finding of this survey reveals that several of the EMR systems in use by SB clinics have the capability to be highly customized to create specific charting workflow. However, many of the institutions using these EMR systems do not know of this capability or do not possess the appropriate resources to create the specific

Table 1
Functionality of a sample of EMR systems used by SB clinics throughout the United States

EMR Functions	Eclipsys Sunrise Ambulatory Care Manager	EPICcare	NextGen EMR	Cerner Powerchart Office/Powerworks EMR	GE Centricity EMR
Alerts—notification of important issues	x	x	x	—	x
Customized templates for documenting specialty specific content	x	x	x	x	—
Image capability with links to scanned files, images, and other media	x	x	x	x	x
Voice recognition compatible	—	x	—	x	x
Evaluation and management coding—automated billing codes for office visits	x	x	x	—	x
Internal messaging—allows staff members to communicate with one another	—	x	—	—	—
Can be used on wireless devices, such as a smart phone	—	x	—	—	—
Can interface with patient portal	x	x	x	x	—
Role-Based security	x	x	x	x	x
Appointments or scheduling	x	x	x	—	x
Electronic prescribing	x	x	x	—	x
Web portal enabled	x	x	—	—	x
Outcomes generator tools	—	x	x	—	x
Interface with other systems	x	x	x	x	x

charting capabilities they need particular to SB clinics. In the latter case, resources such as technical expertise, time, and finances are lacking as indicated in the clinics' survey responses.

Many of the EMRs use narrative text to record much of the clinical information gathered, such as medications or portions of the patient history. Although, in some cases, this may simplify the entry of clinical information, use of narrative text can complicate the retrieval of data. Whether currently using an EMR system or not, 15 out of 16 responding clinics have developed their own mechanisms for data retrieval by using electronic spreadsheets and other electronic database management systems such as Microsoft Access, Filemaker Pro, or SQL Server in place of or in addition to the EMR. Duplicate data entry generates extra time and work on the part of clinic staff, leads to redundancies, and requires additional efforts for maintaining data integrity and security.

Clinicians responding to this survey also indicated that the EMRs being used lack the functionality of sending reminders or alerts for the performance of clinical or administrative tasks. For example, many wanted to receive alerts when a patient's next visit is due or a reminder when laboratory results were outstanding after a certain amount of time had lapsed. Alerts such as these could increase the efficiency in providing continuity of care for patients and ensuring that follow-up care in provided in a timely and consistent manner.

A report by KLAS Enterprises, LLC, an objective evaluator of health care technology and software, reports that significant gaps still exist in several functional areas for EMRs, including tools to generate reports from EMR data, patient access to medical records, and the ability to share key clinical data with other systems.[23] The federal government intends to implement criteria for "meaningful use" of EMR systems in 2011 to determine who will receive Medicare and Medicaid incentives under the American Recovery and Reinvestment Act.[24] During stage one, the Centers for Medicare and Medicaid Services has defined meaningful use objectives under the following general topics:

- Improving quality, safety, efficiency, and care coordination
- Reducing health disparities
- Engaging patients and their families
- Ensuring adequate privacy and security protections of personal health information.[24]

The meaningful use criteria will subsequently be revised in 2013 and again in 2015. At the time of this writing, the meaningful use criteria are still being debated. The implementation of this rule will likely have a profound effect on the EMRs being used.

IMPLEMENTATION OF THE SB EMR

The SB EMR will not replace EMRs currently in use at different institutions, nor is it intended to be the sole charting system that will meet meaningful use guidelines. The SB EMR is a data collection tool that provides for the longitudinal collection of demographic, interventions, and outcomes data, but it is not intended to provide functionality that is necessary to conduct all aspects of a clinic visit in a paperless way. For example, at the University of Pittsburgh Medical Center's (UPMC) adult SB clinic, the EpicCare EMR allows clinicians to enter orders electronically, print prescriptions or transmit them directly to pharmacies, communicate with other clinicians through electronic messages and letters, and submit bills and associated diagnosis codes. Through a separate web-based personal health record portal called UPMC Healthtrak, patients can view portions of their EMR, order refills for their medications, submit questions to clinicians, and request appointments.

The SB EMR, although not intended to replace EMRs in use locally, is intended to augment the data collection systems being used. At UPMC, for example, the templates in EpicCare that drive the structure of the nurse and physician notes are unique to the SB population. The history and physical examination section contains fields for medical conditions and findings that are unique to the SB population and the electronic note can easily be filled out by mouse clicks, small amounts of typing, or dictation. However, information is recorded in free-text prose by ICD codes, and although the notes are archived and searchable, mining those notes for specific data or fields requires time and effort. The SB EMR can augment this data collection system by recording information by choosing data from a pick list or entering in a fixed field much like data are recorded in spreadsheets, which can then be exported and viewed for clinical or research purposes.

Tracking and reminders will be possible with the SB EMR. Tracking visit due dates, what laboratory testing needs to be ordered, and what laboratory results are outstanding will be possible. It will also be possible to track supplies used for bowel, bladder, and wound care and the types of assistive devices that are in use or have been used such as wheelchairs and braces.

Embedded in the SB EMR are hundreds of data fields (variables) that can be recorded. Twenty patient registry variables have been identified as important variables that will be collected by nine clinics in the United States as part of a CDC-funded project:

1. Education
2. Employment
3. Health insurance
4. Marital status
5. Number of SB clinic visits in the last 12 months
6. Head circumference
7. Arm span, standing height, recumbent length
8. Weight
9. Functional level of lesion
10. Neurosurgery
11. Urology surgery
12. Gastrointestinal surgery
13. Skin surgery
14. Ear, nose, or throat surgery
15. Orthopedic procedures
16. Respiratory
17. Bowel management
18. Bladder management
19. Skin integrity
20. Method of mobility.

These variables were chosen as the most likely to yield reliable and meaningful data at the outset of this new process. As the task of data collection matures, the use of the SB EMR is intended to serve as the body of information that, over time, may be included as registry data. The authors view this system of data management as an organized system that uses observational study methods to collect uniform data (clinical and other) to evaluate specified outcomes for the population of people affected by SB.[25]

The SB EMR facilitates the following for its users:

- Replacement of antiquated systems of record keeping and tracking to improve the efficiency of multidisciplinary management of these complex patients
- Enhanced quality and availability of data for clinical use and research
- Increased likelihood of data sharing for national or international studies and collaborations due to the use of standardized terminologies
- Improved patient care through the comparison of care delivered and outcomes realized.

Associated with the SB EMR is a commercially available report writer application, eWebReports by Exago Incorporated, which supports individual clinics in the following ways to allow not only "power users," but also the "casual user," to easily design and execute reports.[26] The New Report Wizard is designed to walk users through all of the required steps in creating a new report, from designing the layout, to selecting filters and sort sequencers, to selecting the output mode (eg, Excel, HTML, PDF, RTF). Some of the features of eWebReports:

- Creation of a single report containing multiple one-to-many relationships
- Creation of fully formatted Excel workbooks (not just CSV files), with user-designed format in an Excel-like grid. This eliminates the guesswork of placing data in the correct cells
- Provision of the ability to design a report and associate a field on the design screen with a PDF form field; upon report execution, the qualifying data is merged into the PDF form.

FUTURE DIRECTIONS

Using a SB-specific, web-based EMR system is expected to provide for consistency in the capture and coding of clinical data to allow for ease of information retrieval across institutions. The clinics who are currently participating in the National Spina Bifida Registry Project have the option of using the SB EMR. In the near future, this web-based SB EMR will be available to clinics nationally to implement in conjunction with current systems used by their institution.

Studies to determine the usability of the SB EMR should be performed to inform and improve upon its functions as the end users (clinicians) provide feedback throughout the implementation process. Simultaneously, another web site developed by the CDC, titled "Preparations," is being launched via a web-based tool developed by the Spina SBA to assist with the transition process for persons with SB. This life-course transition tool has developed pathways for three domains: (1) self-management or health; (2) personal and social relationships; and (3) education or employment support. This web-based Transition Preparation Checklist will provide key developmental milestones in each of these three domains and offer assessment tools, intervention strategies, and patient or caregiver educational materials.[9] In the near future, the SB EMR will be modified to include the Preparation for Adulthood Life course model integrating the Preparations content. This will provide the developmental milestone assessment prompts and suggested tips and resources or interventions that may not typically be considered during usual clinic visits. In addition to serving as a prompting mechanism for the life-course transition process for persons affected by SB, a record will be readily available regarding the assessment, the recommended interventions, and a follow-up reminder to determine and document how successful the implemented interventions were. Such a record could be used to determine the effectiveness of interventions as well as their acceptance by families. Eventual integration of this transition model into the SB EMR will streamline entry and retrieval of data important for the care of persons with SB. With these two tools working in synchrony, many of the desired functions clinicians express in maximizing the benefits of electronic resources may be realized.

REFERENCES

1. White P. Essential components of programs for transition to adulthood. Rev Rhum Engl Ed 1997;64:198S–9S.
2. White P. Future expectations: adolescents with rheumatic diseases and their transition into adulthood. Br J Rheumatol 1996;35:80–3.
3. Sands DJ, Wehmeyer ML. Self-determination across the lifespan: independence and choice for people with disabilities. Baltimore (MD): Paul H. Brookes; 1996. p. 67.
4. Brown J. Orthopaedic care of children with spina bifida: you've come a long way, baby! Orthop Nurs 2001;20:51–8.
5. Dillon C, Davis B, Duquay S, et al. Longevity of patients with myelomeningocele. Eur J Pediatr Surg 2000;10:33–9.
6. Hunt B, Oakeshott P, Kerry S. Link between the CSF shunt and achievement in adults with spina bifida. J Neurol Neurosurg Psychiatr 1999;67:591–5.
7. Wang LY, Paulozzi LJ. Survival of infants with spina bifida: a population study, 1979–94. Paediatr Perinat Epidemiol 2001;15(4):373–8.
8. Liptak G. Evidence-based practice in spina bifida: developing a research agenda. The Spina Bifida Association of America: Washington, DC; 2003. p. 9–10.
9. Thibadeau J, Zabel TA, Fairman AD, et al. Preparation for adult participation. The future is now: First World Congress on Spina Bifida Research and Care. The Spina Bifida Association of America: Orlando (FL); 2009. p. 15–8.
10. Alriksson-Schmidt A, Swanson M, Thibadeau J. The National Spina Bifida Program, 52nd Annual Meeting of the Society for Research into Hydrocephalus and Spina Bifida. The Spina Bifida Association of America: Providence (RI); 2008. p. 11–4.
11. Kohn LT, Corrigan JM, Donaldson MS. To err is human: building a safer health system. Washington, DC: Institute of Medicine (IOM), National Academies Press. Available at: http://books.nap.edu/html/to_err_is_human/reportbrief.pdf. Accessed March 29, 2010.
12. Aspden P, Corrigan JM, Wolcott J, et al. Patient safety: achieving a new standard of care. Washington DC: National Academic Press; 2004. Available at: http://books.nap.edu/openbook.php?record_id=10863. Accessed March 31, 2010.
13. Linder JA, Jun A, Bates DW, et al. Electronic health record use and the quality of ambulatory care in the United States. Arch Intern Med 2007;167(13):1400–5.
14. National Institute of Standards Technology (NIST) Standards and Technical Regulations. Available at: http://ts.nist.gov/Standards/ssd.cfm. Accessed March 31, 2010.
15. Bowman S. Coordination of SNOMED-CT and ICD-10: getting the most out of electronic health record systems. Perspectives in Health Information Management 2005. Available at: http://library.ahima.org/xpedio/groups/public/documents/ahima/bok1_027179. Accessed March 31, 2010.
16. McDonald CJ, Huff SM, Suico JG, et al. LOINC, a universal standard for identifying laboratory observations: a 5-year update. Clin Chem 2003;49:624–33.

17. National Drug Data File (NDDF) Plus. SanBruno (CA): First Databank, Inc. National Drug Data File (NDDF) Plus [cited 2008 Sep 28]. Available at: http://www.firstdatabank.com/products/nddf/. Accessed March 29, 2010.
18. U.S. National Library of Medicine. SNOMED CT to rule based mapping to support reimbursement. Available at: http://www.nih.gov/research/umls/mapping_projects_reimburse. Accessed March 9, 2010.
19. Kohane I, Greenspun P, Fackler J, et al. Building national electronic medical record systems via the World Wide Web. J Am Med Inform Assoc 1996;3: 191–207.
20. Baker JR, Cruidder SO, Riske B, et al. A model for a regional system of care to promote the health and well-being of people with rare chronic genetic disorders. Am J Public Health 2005;95(11):1910–6.
21. Schechter MS, Margolis P. Improving subspecialty healthcare: lessons from cystic fibrosis. J Pediatr 2005;147(3):295–301.
22. Walker J, Pan E, Johnston D, et al. The value of health care information exchange and interoperability. Health Aff 2005. Available at: http://www.nlm.nih.gov/csi/walker_interoperability.pdf. Accessed June 25, 2010.
23. KLAS Enterprises, LLC. Ambulatory EMR: on track for meaningful use? Amb EMR Digest 2009. Available at: www.KLASresearch.org. Accessed June 25, 2010.
24. Executive order 13335, incentives for the use of health information technology and establishing the position of the national health information technology coordinator. Washington, DC; 2004. Available at: http://edocket.access.gpo.gov/2004/pdf/04-10024.pdf. Accessed July 5, 2010
25. Gliklich R, Dreyer N. Registries for evaluating patient outcomes: a user's guide. Prepared by Outcome DEcIDE Center. Rockville (MD): Agency for Healthcare Research; 2007.
26. Exago, Inc. eWebReports delivers easy-to-use ad hoc reporting. Available at: http://exagoinc.com. Accessed July 5, 2010.

Physiatrists and Developmental Pediatricians Working Together to Improve Outcomes in Children with Spina Bifida

Mark E. Swanson, MD, MPH[a],*, Brad E. Dicianno, MD[b,c]

KEYWORDS

• Spina bifida • Physiatry • Developmental pediatrics
• Interdisciplinary care

PHYSIATRY

Physical medicine and rehabilitation (PM&R), also known as physiatry, was officially established by the founding of the American Board of PM&R in the United States in 1947.[1] However, its origins date back to ancient times with the use of physical agents and modalities to prevent and treat diseases. Physiatrists, medical practitioners of physiatry, specialize in the treatment of patients of all ages with musculoskeletal injuries, neuromuscular disorders, pain syndromes, and disabilities, and are trained in electrodiagnostic medicine. The rapid expansion of physiatry can be linked to the

The findings and conclusions in this article are those of the authors and do not necessarily represent the official position of the Centers for Disease Control and Prevention.

The opinions expressed are those of the authors, based on their own experience in the clinical fields of developmental pediatrics and physiatry and do not necessarily reflect the position of any professional organizations or opinions of other physicians with similar backgrounds.

[a] Division of Human Development and Disability, National Center on Birth Defects and Developmental Disabilities, Centers for Disease Control and Prevention, Atlanta, GA, USA

[b] Department of Veterans Affairs, Human Engineering Research Laboratories (HERL), VA Pittsburgh Healthcare System, 7180 Highland Drive, 151R-1, Pittsburgh, PA 15206, USA

[c] Adult Spina Bifida Clinic, Department of Physical Medicine and Rehabilitation, University of Pittsburgh Medical Center (UPMC), Kaufmann Medical Building, Suite 202, 3471 5th Avenue, Pittsburgh, PA 15213, USA

* Corresponding author.

E-mail address: cfu9@cdc.gov

Pediatr Clin N Am 57 (2010) 973–981

doi:10.1016/j.pcl.2010.07.016

0031-3955/10/$ – see front matter. Published by Elsevier Inc.

pediatric.theclinics.com

wars of the twentieth century when evidenced-based rehabilitative strategies were needed to address war casualties.

Physiatrists treat patients in outpatient clinics as well as in acute and subacute inpatient settings. The physiatrist manages specific medical problems of the patient and serves as a team leader, directing a comprehensive rehabilitation care plan that involves other clinicians including physical therapists (PTs) and occupational therapists (OTs), speech language pathologists, nurses, social workers, orthotists, nutritionists, rehabilitation counselors, neuropsychologists, rehabilitation engineers, and others whose main goal is to restore and preserve independent functioning using a team-based approach.

The overall goal of a physiatrist is to promote health and wellness while fostering independence in self-management, communication, and mobility. The physiatrist's ultimate recommendations are based on the patient's own goals and those of caregivers as well as the patient's home and community environments. Treatment plans for a particular problem are not algorithmic in nature, but rather tailored to the individual and the life roles that they fill.

Physiatrists are an essential member of the team of physicians associated with spina bifida (SB) clinics. However, for those who do not have access to a multidisciplinary SB clinic, physiatry may be an ideal medical home for the patient because a physiatrist can act as a team leader and organize the care being provided by multiple specialists in the community.

Although physicians completing a residency in PM&R are trained in pediatric and adult rehabilitation, additional training through fellowships is possible. Pediatric PM&R fellowships are available that can include further training in care of children with disabilities such as SB.

DEVELOPMENTAL PEDIATRICS

The specialty of developmental pediatrics has long been recognized. In the 1960s, pediatricians and child neurologists began to specialize in seeing children with a variety of impairments, including cerebral palsy and intellectual disability (then termed mental retardation). A strong impetus for focused and interdisciplinary care came from the Kennedy family's expressed desire to improve the lives of people with intellectual disability. Federal funding of interdisciplinary centers (university affiliated facilities, the predecessors of many current University Centers of Excellence in Developmental Disabilities) gave universities a physical setting where children could be evaluated by university-based academic physicians, therapists, and other health professionals. Most of the early physician-specialists had been trained in pediatrics and child neurology, but the focus on child development spawned training programs in what became known as developmental pediatrics.

Children's behavior was recognized as an integral part of general pediatric practice in the 1960s. As more and more children with psychosocial problems, termed the new morbidity[2] were recognized, the general pediatrician faced the prospect of being overwhelmed by the time and intensity demands of these children. Child psychiatry was a natural referral destination for children with more severe behaviors, but clearly there have never been enough of this specialty (5000 in 2003) to handle the volume of children identified with mental health problems (7–10 million children in 2003).[3] Although remaining an important part of general pediatrics, academic leaders (including Haggerty and Friedman) led a movement to develop a subspecialty of developmental pediatrics.[3] In an effort to recognize the behavioral and neurologic orientation of developmental pediatrics, the American Board of Pediatrics (ABP) has

2 subspecialties: developmental-behavioral pediatrics and neurodevelopmental disabilities. Each has their own certifying examination. Many physicians have both certifications; of those choosing one, more have opted for the developmental-behavioral designation, a reflection of the larger number of developmental-behavioral pediatrics fellowship opportunities. As in all of pediatrics, the ABP has a Maintenance of Certification (MOC) process in place to ensure that developmental pediatricians sustain skills through clinical practice, quality control, continuing education, and written test performance.

Training for both of the developmental pediatrics subspecialty certifications is currently 3 years of fellowship training after pediatric residency, although many current board-certified specialist programs began in 2001, based on a combination of postresidency training and clinical practice experience. Because of the breadth of clinical issues faced, fellowship programs inevitably have areas of emphasis but must cover training in all areas.

Developmental pediatricians assess the development and behavior of children in the context of the child's overall health and the environment in which the child lives. Areas of assessment include language, motor, attention, cognitive, and social. Clinical impressions are confirmed by formal testing done by other professionals. Interpretation of school and parent questionnaires and other input are part of the developmental pediatrician's responsibilities. The end of an assessment is a profile of the child's functioning in all relevant domains. An intervention plan can include recommendations for further assessment by health and other professionals; behavioral intervention by parents, school, and mental health professionals; use of psychotropic and other medications; and a follow-up visit. Developmental pediatricians communicate with education professionals as part of the follow-up process.

INTERDISCIPLINARY CARE OF THE CHILD WITH SPINA BIFIDA

Pediatric-oriented teams have long served children with SB. The roles of nursing, physical therapy, occupational therapy, speech language pathology, psychology, social work, nutrition, and other disciplines are critical for the effective function of these teams. This article describes the role of the generalist physician (physiatrist or developmental pediatrician) who can unite the work of these disciplines with that of surgical specialists (neurosurgeons, urologists, and orthopedists) to provide holistic, comprehensive care to children with SB.

The developmental pediatrician looks after the developmental, general medical, and behavioral needs of the growing child. Working with therapists, nurses, and social workers, this part of the interdisciplinary team takes a holistic approach to try to normalize the child's development and function at home and school. Those issues with a strong developmental theme throughout the child's life are addressed by this group: school performance, social skills, sexuality, to name a few.

In the 1990s, clinicians began to appreciate that rehabilitation medicine care was needed to supplement the more traditional interdisciplinary care provided by pediatricians and other health professionals. The heightened expectation for people with SB to function in their homes and communities drove this need for rehabilitation expertise.[4] Children with SB had attendant needs to monitor this progress in the interdisciplinary clinic as they developed. Physiatry's emphasis on function was critical in the planning for independent living and participation. The introduction of the International Classification of Functioning, Health, and Disability (ICF)[5] has reinforced this notion by offering language and terminology to describe the outcomes (participation) as well as the process (interaction of impairment with environment). Although there is not an absolute dichotomy between developmental pediatrics and physiatry, each brings its own focus to the interdisciplinary care of children with SB. Child development, behavior, anticipatory guidance, and connection to educational services are all strengths of the developmental pediatrician. Measuring and promoting function, all aimed at increased activities and participation are major contributions of physiatry.

The next sections describe the different contributions made by the 2 disciplines to the care of children with SB regarding specific issues.

Health Self-management

Developmental pediatricians are particularly oriented towards involving families in monitoring their child's condition in the context of family dynamics and normal child development. The stress of chronic illness on family members and the child may be substantial. It requires that the child and family's coping skills be monitored carefully and regularly. Acquiring health self-management skills, beginning in early childhood, requires an understanding of how the child is developing in motor and cognitive skills, as well as socially and emotionally. Helping parents let go of their tendency to maintain care for the child whom they perceive as vulnerable is an important task of health care providers. Letting the adolescent schedule appointments, directing questions to the adolescent during clinic visits, and encouraging the adolescent to manage medication refills are examples of strategies to promote self-management for adolescents. Physiatrists reinforce these same behaviors in children and families in their care.

Physical Fitness and Activity

Lifelong impairments in mobility present challenges for exercise and have resulted in alarming rates of obesity in patients with SB.[6] Adolescents and young adults tend to be physically inactive, with poor aerobic fitness and high body fat.[7] Developmental pediatricians have an orientation to normal growth that should encourage them to monitor weight gain, and its relation to nutrition and physical activity. Because nutrition is the key to weight gain, the consulting nutritionist is an invaluable member of the team. Physiatry may take the lead on choice of activities that will burn calories and minimize risk of overuse strain and injury.

Physiatric interventions include counseling and customization of creative diet and home exercise plans that use available resources and overcome barriers caused by cost, transportation, motivation, or physical inaccessibility. Constructing a team of support from caregivers, trainers, nutritionists, PTs, and/or OTs is helpful.

Neuromuscular Disorders

Musculoskeletal disorders are also common. Repetitive strain injuries, nerve entrapments, orthopedic deformities, back pain, and contractures may require conservative management by a physiatrist either after surgery or when surgical options are limited.[8] Although most individuals with SB have a lower motor neuron injury and thus do not have spasticity, increased tone can emerge for those with tethered cord syndrome.[8] Treatment is indicated when increased tone causes pain, barriers to self-care or hygiene, or when impending contracture poses a threat to optimal function or joint position. Physiatry approaches include physical or occupational therapy, oral medications, botulinum toxin, neurolysis, serial casting, and wheelchair positioning, but surgical options such as implantable pumps may be indicated in severe cases.

Mobility (Including Assistive Devices/Durable Medical Equipment)

Approximately 60% of individuals with SB use assistive technologies (AT) for mobility including manual, power-assisted, and power wheelchairs.[9] Physiatrists specialize in

AT prescription and can help patients with SB and their families navigate the difficult world of insurance claims to obtain needed equipment. An evaluation for AT should include a physiatrist, a PT or OT, a supplier, and sometimes a rehabilitation engineer. Physiatrists also work closely with vocational rehabilitation services and may consult rehabilitation counselors to aid their patients in obtaining financial support for AT needed for education or employment. Many individuals may also need other AT such as computer access equipment or mobility equipment to meet their school or work goals.

Developmental pediatrics includes the dimension of suggesting activities for which mobility might be needed: service organizations, school functions (academic and extracurricular), recreation, and age-appropriate social functions.

Pain

Through familiarity with treatment of neuromuscular pain, the physiatrist is critically important in determining options, initiating interventions, and monitoring results of pain management plans. Acute and chronic pain can pose a significant threat to independent function and quality of life. Treatment approaches are often multimodal, including psychology, medications, interventional injections and procedures, PT, OT, and many integrative, complementary, and alternative approaches. The pediatrician can help with issues of adherence by parents and patients to routines, awareness of exacerbating and ameliorating factors in the home or school environment and side effects of treatment. The pediatrician can ensure that plans are developmentally appropriate and that monitoring and reporting of interventions are shared by the child and family.

Bowel Management

Most children with SB have bowel problems, including constipation and incontinence. Neurologic deficits lead to incontinence; low abdominal muscle tone, lack of dietary fiber, and lack of physical activity contribute to constipation.[10] Bowel management is a critical component of a plan to manage skin care and to promote socialization. The pediatrician lends perspective to normal development of bowel continence and the health and social consequences of encopresis and impaction. Physiatrists will tailor a bowel program to each individual, using a combination of medications, timed toileting programs, and diet.[11] Surgical procedures are available for refractory cases. Nurses may take a lead role in teaching patients and caregivers how to carry out a bowel program.

Bladder Management

Many individuals with SB experience incontinence and urinary tract infections (UTIs) as a result of neurogenic bladder. Urodynamic testing can identify a wide spectrum of abnormalities, including upper and lower motor neuron types of bladder and urethral dysfunction.[12,13] A physiatrist or pediatrician may be involved in the basic treatment of neurogenic bladder, which includes oral medications[14] or clean intermittent catheterization (CIC). In many cases management by a urologist is necessary for surgical or interventional procedures. Asymptomatic bacteriuria in those using a CIC program does not typically require antibiotic therapy unless reflux into the ureters is present,[15] but treatment of true infections is necessary to prevent renal damage and sepsis. Several measures can be used in the prevention of UTI.[16]

The developmental pediatrician lends expertise in decisions about the child's role in managing the CIC program. With other team members (psychology, nursing, social work), the developmental pediatrician can gauge the family's readiness to begin

CIC and then oversee the child taking increasing responsibility for this process. The developmental pediatrician can share in management of UTI with the primary care pediatrician and the urologist.

Wounds and Skin Care

The causes of wounds in the SB population are often multifactorial, related to many issues such as nutritional status, pressure, shear, moisture, and even burns.[17] Vigilant skin self-inspection and care is fundamental to prevention of breakdown or complications from already open wounds. Wound care including nutritional support, pressure relief techniques, treatment of incontinence, sharp and enzymatic debridement, wound gels and barrier ointments, and dressings are conservative management tools that physiatrists implement. Serious wounds may require surgical or infectious disease consultation.

Sexuality and Personal Relationships

A comprehensive evaluation for any adolescent or adult with SB should also include an assessment of sexuality. People with SB rarely get sexual education from physicians,[18] but most individuals with SB desire more information on fertility and sexuality.[19]

These 2 issues are inextricably linked and should be addressed jointly by clinicians. Personal relationships begin in early childhood and progress to emotional and physical intimacy only after a long series of developmental steps.[20] The developmental pediatrician should monitor development of friendships during childhood and anticipate the sexual awakening that occurs with puberty. Because many children with SB may experience puberty that precedes their emotional maturity, clinicians need to be sensitive to the internal tension (normal for typical children, perhaps enhanced for children with SB[21]) caused by this dichotomy. The developmental pediatrician should lead efforts to track how a child is doing in relationship development and encourage families to allow for the kind of social experiences that will promote such development. The pediatrician must allow the parent to find the delicate balance between safe and developmentally appropriate social experiences for the child with mobility limitations. Physiatry can lend expertise in movement, positioning, and sensation to the child learning about function and self-management of sexual organs, bowel, and bladder.

Physiatrists are trained to understand reproductive issues and how they relate to spinal cord dysfunction and can be a valuable educative source for patients on this topic.

Education

Developmental pediatricians have special expertise in assessing the educational needs and proposing interventions. Using input from psychologists, speech and language pathologists, and special educators, the developmental pediatrician should provide input into the individualized education plan (IEP). Their experience in interacting with the school, for both assessment and planned interventions, should support the parent and child in determining the best IEP. Other complicating behaviors (inattention, depression, acting out) can be assessed and followed by the developmental pediatrician. If the child does not qualify for special education and an IEP, the developmental pediatrician can help parents request a 504 assessment, which could also yield an individualized plan.[22]

Preparation for Employment

Developmental pediatricians know the adolescent's academic potential and can discuss career opportunities with the adolescent and parents. The developmental pediatrician should monitor the required transition plan if the child has an IEP and also monitor and encourage the development of age-appropriate home responsibilities, which can indicate an adolescent's readiness to take on more adult responsibilities. The physiatrist should take the lead on the accommodations that need to be made for the adolescent to have volunteer and work experience, which may include transportation to the work site and technological accommodations within the work place (for mobility, communication, or computer access). Job coaching and mentoring can be directed by either the developmental pediatrician or physiatrist. When services and funding from the state's Vocational Rehabilitation Department need to be accessed, the physiatrist often has the best experience to handle this. Physiatry's orientation to restoring functional skills (driving, mobility) in people with spinal cord injury could be invaluable in establishing similar skills in adolescents with SB.

Working Together

Developmental pediatricians excel at the developmental, behavioral, and educational aspects of SB care. Their training in normal development helps guide monitoring of the progress children make in many of the important domains described in the Life Course Model for SB (see the article by Swanson in this issue). Social and behavioral adjustment is monitored using parent interviews and administration of a formal behavioral rating instrument (with the aid of psychologists). School readiness and watchful anticipation for learning disabilities, language problems, and other executive function disorders are monitored with information from schools and language therapists. Co-occurring problems with sleep, attention, and depression suit the training of the developmental pediatrician. The developmental pediatrician can also help implement plans for shunt management, bowel and bladder management, and skin care that may be initiated by other professionals. When a primary care pediatrician is not strongly involved, due attention to coordination of care and linkage to community resources may be the responsibility of the developmental pediatrician.

Physiatrists play a key role in treating conditions such as skin breakdown, neurogenic bowel and bladder, and musculoskeletal conditions, while focusing on how these conditions affect independence and function. A physiatrist aims to improve health and wellness through promotion of activity and independent mobility and to lessen the effect of secondary disabling medical conditions. The physiatrist views the patient as a whole, rather than an organ system, and a person within the broader context of their environment and life roles. With this view, and by acting as a coordinator of many disciplines, the physiatrist can help to ensure that the patient's care plan is suited to promote the patient's goals and the highest level of independent functioning possible.

SUMMARY

Based on the experience of 2 physicians from physiatry and developmental pediatrics, this article proposes a framework for improving care and outcomes for children with SB. The combined skills of physiatrists and developmental pediatricians, along with other disciplines, can form the ideal team to manage the complex issues faced by this population. The developmental pediatrician is best suited for directing care for younger children through the elementary and middle school years, during which time behavioral and educational issues are prominent. As the child assumes more responsibility for self-management in adolescence, the physiatrist is ideally suited to providing major clinical input that improves functional outcomes. The addition of the discipline of physiatry to traditional, developmentally oriented pediatric interdisciplinary teams can add the much needed dimensions of activity and participation, and improve functional outcomes at the adult level by encouraging activities in adolescence that lead to full participation in adulthood.

REFERENCES

1. Opitz JL, Folz TJ, Gelfman R, et al. The history of physical medicine and rehabilitation as recorded in the diary of Dr. Frank Krusen: part 1. Gathering Momentum (the Years Before 1942). Arch Phys Med Rehabil 1997;78:442–4.
2. Haggerty RJ, Roghman KJ, Pless IB. Child health and the community. New York: John Wiley; 1975. p. 94–5.
3. Haggerty RJ, Friedman SB. History of developmental-behavioral pediatrics. J Dev Behav Pediatr 2003;24:S1–17.
4. Kinsman SL, Levey E, Ruffing V, et al. Beyond multidisciplinary care: a new conceptual model for spina bifida. Eur J Pediatr Surg 2000;10(Suppl 1):35–8.
5. Lollar DJ, Simeonsson RJ. Diagnosis to function: classification for children and youths. J Dev Behav Pediatr 2005;26(4):323–30.
6. Dosa NP, Foley JT, Eckrich M, et al. Obesity across the lifespan among persons with spina bifida. Disabil Rehabil 2009;31(11):914–20.
7. Buffart LM, Roebroeck ME, Rol M, et al. Triad of physical activity, aerobic fitness and obesity in adolescents and young adults with myelomeningocele. J Rehabil Med 2008;40(1):70–5.
8. Dicianno BE, Kurowski BG, Yang JM, et al. Rehabilitation and medical management of the adult with spina bifida. Am J Phys Med Rehabil 2008;87(12):1027.
9. Dicianno BE, Gaines A, Collins DM, et al. Mobility, assistive technology use, and social integration among adults with spina bifida. Am J Phys Med Rehabil 2009; 88(7):533.
10. Sullivan PB. Gastrointestinal disorders in children with neurodevelopmental disabilities. Dev Disabil Res Rev 2008;14(2):128–36.
11. Bischoff A, Levitt MA, Bauer C, et al. Treatment of fecal incontinence with a comprehensive bowel management program. J Pediatr Surg 2009;44(6): 1278–84.
12. Kessler TM, Lackner J, Kiss G, et al. Predictive value of initial urodynamic pattern on urinary continence in patients with myelomeningocele. Neurourol Urodyn 2006;25(4):361.
13. Sakakibara R, Hattori T, Uchiyama T, et al. Uroneurological assessment of spina bifida cystica and occulta. Neurourol Urodyn 2003;22(4):328–34.
14. Chancellor MB, Anderson RU, Boone TB. Pharmacotherapy for neurogenic detrusor overactivity. Am J Phys Med Rehabil 2006;85(6):536–45.
15. Ottolini MC, Shaer CM, Rushton HG, et al. Relationship of asymptomatic bacteriuria and renal scarring in children with neuropathic bladders who are practicing clean intermittent catheterization. J Pediatr 1995;127(3):368–72.
16. Biering-Sørensen F. Urinary tract infection in individuals with spinal cord lesion. Curr Opin Urol 2002;12(1):45.
17. Balakrishnan C, Rak TP, Meininger MS. Burns of the neuropathic foot following use of therapeutic footbaths. Burns 1995;21:622–3.
18. Cardenas DD, Topolski TD, White CJ, et al. Sexual functioning in adolescents and young adults with spina bifida. Arch Phys Med Rehabil 2008;89(1):31–5.

19. Sawyer SM, Roberts KV. Sexual and reproductive health in young people with spina bifida. Dev Med Child Neurol 1999;41(10):671–5.
20. Blum RW, Resnick MD, Nelson R, et al. Family and peer issues among adolescents with spina bifida and cerebral palsy. Pediatrics 1991;88(2):280–5.
21. Sawin KJ, Buran CF, Brei TJ, et al. Sexuality issues in adolescents with a chronic neurological condition. J Perinat Educ 2002;11(1):22–34.
22. American Academy of Pediatrics: The pediatrician's role in development and implementation of an individual education plan (IEP) and/or an individual family service plan (IFSP). Pediatrics 1999;104(1):124–7.

Approaches to Transition in Other Chronic Illnesses and Conditions

Cecily L. Betz, PhD, RN[a,b],*

KEYWORDS

- Transition • Cystic fibrosis • Spina bifida
- Congenital heart disease • Childhood cancer
- Life Course Model

This article provides an overview of the strategic efforts to promote health care transition planning for people with cystic fibrosis, congenital heart disease (CHD), and spina bifida, and survivors of childhood cancer. Prevalence and life expectancy data are presented, in addition to data on long-term outcomes as background information for the need for health care transition planning efforts. Efforts to improve the provision of transition services provided to these groups of youth with chronic conditions and their families are compared and contrasted with efforts under development for youth with spina bifida. With a description of varied approaches, this article intends to portray these efforts as models that could be replicated for other groups of youth with chronic illnesses and conditions. The Life Course Model for spina bifida detailed in other articles in this journal serves as a reference point for efforts in other chronic conditions.

Adults with childhood-acquired chronic conditions and their families have long recognized the need for a system of care that facilitates their transfer from pediatric to adult health services and other programs that support their transition into adulthood. The longstanding angst and frustration they experienced for decades finally reached a critical mass, and their collective voices were finally heard about addressing their needs. In contrast to the shortened life expectancy and tumultuous and uncertain course of children born with chronic conditions just a few decades ago, the life expectancy of this group of children now extends into adulthood, with 90% expected to

[a] Department of Pediatrics, Keck School of Medicine, University of Southern California, Los Angeles, CA, USA
[b] USC Center of Excellence in Developmental Disabilities, Childrens Hospital Los Angeles, 4650 Sunset Boulevard, MS# 53, Los Angeles, CA 90027, USA
* USC Center of Excellence in Developmental Disabilities, Childrens Hospital Los Angeles, 4650 Sunset Boulevard, MS# 53, Los Angeles, CA 90027.
E-mail address: CLBetz@aol.com

Pediatr Clin N Am 57 (2010) 983–996
doi:10.1016/j.pcl.2010.07.017   **pediatric.theclinics.com**
0031-3955/10/$ – see front matter © 2010 Elsevier Inc. All rights reserved.

survive to the second decade of life.[1] As evidenced by this recognition, pediatric specialty and subspecialty organizations and governmental agencies are advancing practice principles for health care transition planning.[2] Likewise, interdisciplinary pediatric researchers are beginning to seriously tackle the issues associated with health care transition planning through developing psychometrically credible instruments to test the effectiveness of interventions in improving outcomes for youth with chronic conditions.[2–4]

Several impressive developments reflect improvements in the life expectances of children born with chronic conditions. The mean survival of adults with cystic fibrosis is 37.4 years, and the life expectancy for adults with sickle cell disease is 42 years for men and 48 years for women.[5–7] Although the number of adults with childhood-acquired chronic conditions is difficult to estimate, reliable approximations of these numbers have been offered. There are an estimated 300,000 adult survivors of childhood acquired cancer, and the Adult Congenital Heart Association estimates that there are 1.8 million adult survivors of CHD.[8] Although estimations of the number of adults with spina bifida have not been reported, an estimated 75% of children with spina bifida survive into early adulthood.[9]

This article compares and contrasts the profile of efforts undertaken to improve the provision of transition services provided to selected groups of youth with chronic conditions and their families. The groups of chronically ill youth presented in this article are those with cystic fibrosis and CHD, and survivors of childhood cancer. Discussion of each of these chronic conditions begins with a brief profile of demographic data as it pertains to prevalence, rates of mortality and morbidity, and life expectancy. This section is followed by concise summary of data on adult educational, employment, and psychosocial outcomes. Descriptions of the efforts to improve transition services and adult outcomes are provided and compared and contrasted with the efforts under development for youth with spina bifida. Other articles in this issue can be referred to as appropriate for additional discussion of content areas pertaining to youth with spina bifida. The description of systematic efforts will also reveal areas for future development and their implications for practice and research.

The acquisition of self-management skills essential to fostering positive health outcomes and self-reliance in living with a chronic condition are emphasized. The newly developed Web-based resource for families and youth with spina bifida is designed to comprehensively provide information and resources that can be accessed to achieve the goals of health care transition planning. The spina bifida Web-based resource is an example of a tool that provides condition-specific information for self-management, and also information on general management that is not unique to spina bifida, because all children who have a chronic condition need to learn these general self-management skills.

These general self-management skills that must be learned to the greatest extent possible by all children and youth who have chronic conditions include making care appointments, ordering medications, communicating with the health provider, and managing sexuality/puberty issues. Examples of other general self-management behaviors are practicing good oral health habits; regular exercise; healthy eating and cooking; avoidance of high-risk behaviors that are detrimental to one's chronic condition and health, such as alcohol and drugs use; and enrollment in an adult health insurance plan.

The following section presents information on the unified national efforts that have been undertaken to foster health care transition planning for youth with CHD. Prevalence data and findings from studies examining outcomes of adults with CHD are offered.

YOUTH WITH CONGENITAL HEART DISEASE

Recent estimates of survival rates indicate that approximately 85% of infants born with CHD will survive into adulthood. The estimates of adults with CHD in the United States are difficult to calculate accurately because no national registry of adults with CHD exists, unlike other industrialized countries, such as England, with national health care registries, although these registries also have their limitations.[10,11] Experts estimate that the number of adults with CHD currently vary up to 1.8 million, more than the number of children with CHD. These estimates represent a profound change in the profile of individuals living with CHD and the system of care needed to respond to this new requirement for services.[8,12–14] Proportionally, there are three adults with CHD for every child with CHD.[12,14] Among the adults with CHD, 80,000 are projected to have severe CHD.[12,14] Now, with the extended survival of individuals with CHD, most deaths occur in adulthood rather than in childhood.[10]

Adults with CHD require life-long surveillance.[15] Long-term monitoring is needed to detect and prevent complications associated with arrhythmias, congestive heart failure, premature death, and bacterial endocarditis.[16,17] Several follow-up studies have been conducted to investigate morbidity and mortality and expenditures for services. A study of Belgian adults with CHD found that 20% required hospitalizations for cardiac and noncardiac surgical and medical purposes and their care generated higher cost expenditures compared with the general population. A Canadian study showed that 47% of adults with complex CHD were successfully transferred to adult care.[12] Canadian adults with complex CHD were found to have high rates of hospitalizations and emergency room visits after their transition to adult providers.[12] Other follow-up studies conducted in the United States have reported similar findings.[15]

These and other studies identified barriers to accessing care. The Canadian and United States systems showed a lack of training programs for physicians, service integration between pediatric and adult systems, and trained providers.[18] In the Canadian system, placement on the waiting list also was found to result in service delay.[18] In a study examining access to care, approximately 30% of individuals with moderate to complex heart problems reported lapses with their care. Lack of follow-up occurred for several reasons: (1) patients were told that follow-up was not important (33%), (2) no transfer to an adult provider occurred (23%), (3) patients believed follow-up was not important (19%), (4) lack of insurance (19%), and (5) patients were fearful of hearing bad news (7%).[19] Those who experienced a lapse in care were more likely to require urgent care for their cardiac problem.[19]

As these findings indicate, adults with CHD have significant ongoing needs for care that require constant surveillance and monitoring. Additionally, adults with CHD have higher rates of hospitalization and emergency room visits than the general population. As the results of the study by Yeung and colleagues[19] showed, and anecdotal accounts of clinicians have corroborated, the health literacy of emerging adults is inadequate, resulting in lapses of care, untoward consequences of ignoring cardiac problems, and more serious cardiac problems requiring hospitalization or urgent care. Findings of studies and surveys of professional organizations conclude that access to competent adult health care providers knowledgeable about the long-term care needs of adults with CHD is an ongoing problem.[20–22]

In 2001, the American College of Cardiology (ACC) hosted the 32nd Bethesda Conference, *Care of the Adult with Congenital Heart Disease*,[22] to address the emerging and pressing needs of this new population with CHD to develop and implement a strategic plan for a continuous, ongoing, comprehensive, and specialized system of care for the future. To comprehensively address the range of issues encountered by adults with CHD, five task forces were commissioned to address a specific area of need with an action plan. Each of the five task forces was delegated the responsibility of generating a set of recommendations to address the following thematic areas included in the Bethesda report: (1) the clinical profile of adults with CHD and their unmet needs for services; (2) special health care needs of adults with CHD; (3) workforce educational requirements for the growing population of adults with CHD; (4) a system of care needed for adults with CHD,[23–25] and (5) access to health care and adult services for education, employment, and community living.[20,26]

The guidelines recommended the establishment of regional interdisciplinary centers for treating adults with CHD.[19] Currently 55 centers exist in the United States and 15 in Canada.[12] And estimated 20,000 of adults with CHD are provided services at these centers, which is significantly less than the approximately 1.8 million adults with CHD identified earlier.[15] The significant disparity between the actual numbers of adults with CHD and those served demonstrate the challenges in establishing a system to provide services required by this growing population.[15,21] Currently, no uniform standards of practice have been implemented for treating adults with CHD, resulting in differing services available at each of the centers.

The goal of the recommendations generated by each of the task forces was to develop a long-term strategic plan that would provide the foundation for a system of care to competently address the unique health care needs of adults with CHD. Although the Bethesda recommendations were directed to improve health outcomes of adults with CHD, the intended audience for application was pediatric and adult cardiologists. A legitimate system of care to address the unmet needs for services encountered by adults with CHD is not possible without sufficient numbers of adult cardiologists with specialty training in managing this patient population.

Given the rising numbers of adults living with CHD, the American College of Cardiology Foundation (ACCF) and American Heart Association (AHA) developed guidelines for care of adults with CHD. The most recent version presents the evidence-based medical guidelines. The emphasis of these guidelines is on the medical aspects of care.[19,21]

No formalized program or system of care for transitioning exists in the United States or in Brittan. The initiation of care transfer is not predicated on chronologic age, although experts suggest it should occur somewhere between 12 and 16 years of age; however, a combination of factors, such as emotional maturity, gender, disease status, and family functioning, affect the transfer initiation.[10,21] Although the ACCF/AHA provided guidelines for implementing adult programs, the focus is on promoting medical services. This document also specified service recommendations, including age of transfer, medical summary and transfer of records, and the providers' medical qualifications for care.[21]

An obvious service gap is the lack of a best practice template for health care transition planning. A comprehensive health care transition planning approach incorporates the best practices advocated by the American Academy of Pediatrics (AAP) consensus statement.[2] Best practices include support for a comprehensive, interdisciplinary service approach. An integrated and comprehensive model of care includes not only the needs related to survivorship but an examination of health-related needs pertaining to future employment, psychosocial concerns, exercise, high-risk behaviors, pregnancy and contraception, preventive approaches to minimizing the possibilities of complications such as infectious endocarditis, and need for noncardiac surgeries.

ADULT SURVIVORS OF CHILDHOOD CANCER

Each year approximately 12,400 children and youth are diagnosed with some type of cancer.[27] The advances in treatment of pediatric cancers have improved the survivorship of children diagnosed with cancer; each year, the survival rate for adolescents increases approximately 0.9%.[28,29] Currently, 80% of children diagnosed with cancer survive into adulthood,[30] and there are an estimated 300,000 adult survivors of childhood cancer in United States.[31]

The life expectancy for cancer survivors is on average approximately 10 years less than for the general population, although it varies according to the type of cancer. For example, the life expectancy is reduced by 4 years for individuals diagnosed with kidney tumors and by 17 years for those with Ewing's sarcoma and brain tumors.[32] The survivorship data do not reflect current treatment advances because they are based on patients treated from 20 to 40 years ago.[33]

Major survivorship issues exist pertaining to the occurrence of treatment-related late effects, secondary to the primary cancer diagnosis and the psychosocial ramifications associated with the lived experience of the cancer diagnosis and the late effects. Given these circumstances, experts urge the implementation of a health care transition plan that includes the adoption of a long-term survivorship plan for life-long surveillance.[29] Understanding of the range of potential biopsychosocial late effects and secondary conditions a child or adolescent with cancer may experience will provide a context for developing guidelines of care to address these concerns. As this discussion shows, the guidelines of care reflect the medical best practices recommended by the clinical community. Additional empiric testing is needed to show the effectiveness of care recommended.

The late effects from treatment-related complications associated with radiation, chemotherapy, hematopoietic stem cell transplantation, and surgery have been described as changes in physical appearance (ie, surgical scars, amputations), orthopedic problems (ie, short stature), endocrine dysfunctions (ie, hypo/hyperthyroidism, growth hormone deficiency), neurocognitive deficits (ie, attention deficit–hyperactivity disorder, learning disabilities), pulmonary dysfunction (ie, pulmonary fibrosis, obstructive lung disease), cardiac problems (cardiomyopathy, valvular disease), reproductive dysfunction (ie, premature menopause, ovarian failure, sterility), and second malignant tumors (ie, thyroid, breast cancer).[29,34–36] Childhood cancer survivors are six times more likely to develop a second cancer.[34]

These late-effects are not uncommon, occurring in two of every three survivors.[35] Studies have concluded that cancer survivors originally diagnosed with brain tumors have more serious late effects.[37]

Approximately 75% of cancer survivors will develop a chronic condition by 40 years of age. Nearly 50% are expected to exhibit declines in functional abilities and ability to be physically active.[36] Many of these problems are treatable, such as those associated with endocrine and cardiovascular late effects.[38] The key to treatment is early detection of problems by the survivor's adult primary and specialty care physicians, which are discussed in greater detail later.

Much of the evidence on childhood cancer survivorship has been reported from analyses of Childhood Cancer Survivor Study (CCSS) data. The CCSS is a retrospective ascertained cohort of 20,346 childhood cancer survivors diagnosed before age 21 between January 1, 1970 and December 31, 1986, and 4000 siblings who served as the control group, from 26 participating clinical research centers in the United States and Canada.[39] The data were compiled from survivors of the following cancer groups: leukemia, central nervous system cancers, Hodgkin lymphoma, Wilms' tumor, neuroblastoma, soft tissue sarcoma, and bone tumors. More recently the cohort was expanded to include 5-year survivors diagnosed from January 1, 1987 to December 31, 1999.[40]

An overview of the findings of studies conducted with childhood cancer survivors show the range of late effects. Follow-up studies of cancer survivors that involved measurement of behavioral and psychosocial constructs found that they scored lowered than comparison groups of siblings or matched typical peers.[41,42] CCSS survivors (mean age, 14.8 years; range 12–17 years), in contrast to the comparison group of siblings (mean age, 14.9 years; same range), were more likely to have higher levels of behavioral and social problems in the domains of depression/anxiety symptoms (1.5 times higher) and attention deficits and antisocial behaviors (1.7 times) compared with siblings. Survivors diagnosed with leukemia and central nervous system tumors had more difficulties.[41] Another study reported that one of five survivors had posttraumatic stress disorder, as did parents and siblings.[36] Findings from a study of 103 Greek cancer survivors (mean age, 19.8 years) and their matched peer controls showed that survivors scored lower than the control subjects on measures of social functioning and self-esteem.[42]

Several studies have examined quality of life among childhood cancer survivors. Findings showed that survivor scores were similar to comparison groups in most domains, except physical well-being for which the scores were lower. Lower quality-of-life scores were associated with smaller subgroups of survivors who had the following characteristics: older at diagnosis, longer time since diagnosis, female sex, specific diagnoses (ie, bone and central nervous system tumors), selected personal attributes (ie, low self-esteem), physical symptoms (fatigue), and demographics (ie, socioeconomic status, Hispanic ethnicity).[43,44]

Studies of the academic performance of childhood cancer survivors show that they are at higher risk for academic problems and adverse outcomes. Academic problems include higher rates of special education enrollment, high school dropouts, and learning disabilities. The adverse outcomes associated with academic performance are attributable to learning difficulties that result from treatments effects, which cause declines in executive functioning, memory capacity, processing speed, and visual perceptual skills.[36]

Successful transition to adulthood may be described by the achievement of developmental milestones. These developmental milestones include completion of postsecondary education or training programs for occupational or career purposes, employment, and development of significant relationships (ie, romantic relationships, marriage, long-term partnerships) and starting a family.

Studies investigating employment status of survivors found that rates of full-time employment were 10% to 15% lower than for the typical population. Unemployment rates were considerably higher (20%–50%[32]) for those who underwent radiation treatment, were diagnosed with a brain tumor, were diagnosed at a younger age, and had a chronic medical condition. Unemployment rates were higher for female survivors.[32,45,46]

Outcomes associated with romantic relationships and marriage indicate that survivors experience more challenges compared with the general population. In a study of 60 emerging adult cancer survivors, subjects reported fewer relationships and were more upset when the relationship terminated compared with the control group. Those at higher risk for relationship difficulties were survivors who were older when diagnosed, were exposed to a more rigorous treatment regimen, and reported higher levels of anxiety.[47] Rigorous treatment sequelae can cause physical and cognitive limitations that adversely affect social relationships.

Findings pertaining to marital status have been inconsistent regarding rates of marriage.[39,46] One study suggested that rates of marriage for survivors were comparable to national averages.[46] Other findings show that rates of marriage were lower; one study reported nearly two times lower rates for survivors when compared with their siblings.[36,39] Lower marriage rates were attributed to factors such as the treatment-related effects of short stature, impaired physical functioning, decreased executive function, and memory capacity.

Investigations conducted to examine health care use by survivors show the significant gaps in adult care. In one study, 90% of survivors reported having a primary care provider, and approximately 50% had a complete physical examination in the past year.[46] In another study, clinic nonattendance was associated with survivors who were older, of lower socioeconomic status, noninsured, off treatment for a longer period, and nonwhite.[48] Researchers suggest that low socioeconomic status is a proxy for a greater burden of stress, a high level of competing family demands, and fewer resources available (ie, transportation and child care), which adversely affect the long-term management of survivors.[49]

A systematic review of studies found that survivors had lower rates of smoking, alcohol use, and unprotected sex than the survivor population when compared with siblings and controls. Survivors of higher socioeconomic status were engaged in healthier behaviors. Substance abuse was associated with anxiety about cancer.[50]

Studies have shown health literacy of long-term cancer survivors to be problematic. Findings from one study found that 70% of 121 cancer survivors did not remember receiving information from health care providers about the late effects of treatment.[29] An investigation of Internet use among cancer survivors and their parents found that 90% accessed the Internet; approximately 30% used it to locate answers to unanswered questions after their health care visit (which were unasked for a variety of reasons, such as forgot or uncomfortable asking the question), 50% to obtain health information, and 10% to seek information about late effects.[51]

As the CCSS findings and those from other investigations show, cancer survivors have a range of biopsychosocial needs and problems that require ongoing support and services. Their unmet needs result in unfavorable outcomes indicating problems with successful adaptation to adulthood, including lower rates of employment, academic challenges, and difficulties with social and romantic relationships, and the range of late effects described earlier.

Study findings reveal the lack of transition programs available to support survivors with the transfer to adult health care providers who are knowledgeable about late effects and health risks, and to coordinate this transfer and refer survivors to other adult social, educational, employment programs.[36] This service gap is widespread, even in countries with universal access to health care.[36] System barriers, such as lack of subspecialty providers, lack of knowledge by primary providers, and lack of communication between pediatric and adult providers regarding care, have been cited as contributing to the inconsistencies in follow-up. Preventive strategies must be developed to facilitate early detection and ongoing screening.[34]

In an effort to provide clinical guidelines for health care professionals who provide long-term management for survivors of childhood cancer, the Children's Oncology Group (COG), a national network of more than 200 institutions involved in clinical trials, developed the *Long-term Follow-up Guidelines for Survivors of Childhood, Adolescent, and Young Adult Cancers* (COG LTFU guidelines). The purpose of this resource is to improve the care provided to asymptomatic cancer survivors for ongoing long-term surveillance, early detection, and prevention.[35] The COG LTFU guidelines are intended to be used by practitioners in the development of a survivorship care plan that contains individualized long-term treatment recommendations by pediatric primary care and adult providers after patients are transferred to the adult health care system. The AAP recommendations for long-term management of pediatric cancer survivors based on the COG LTFU guidelines also include health promotion guidelines and prevention recommendations to avoid high-risk behaviors pertaining to tobacco and alcohol use and engage in healthy behaviors. Together these guidelines focus on the medical and health needs of childhood cancer survivors. Guidelines addressing the range of comprehensive needs according to best practice models have not been developed, including those related to self-management.

CYSTIC FIBROSIS

Cystic fibrosis is the most frequently occurring autosomal recessive disease with life-threatening consequences. In the United States, 1 in 3500 newborns is affected. Approximately 30,000 individuals have cystic fibrosis.[52] Early diagnosis and treatment, ongoing effective home and self-management, and lesser disease severity are associated with longer life expectancy.[53] Treatment improvements have resulted in reduced mortality rates and increased life expectancy.[53,54] Currently, the life expectancy of an individual with cystic fibrosis is 37.4 years.[5] Recent data showing that the percentage of individuals with cystic fibrosis alive at 19 years of age rose from 88% of individuals born between 1985 to 1989 to 92% of individuals born between 1990 to 1994 indicate the improved survival rates.[5] The life expectancy for individuals with cystic fibrosis is projected to steadily increase from the high 30s for those born in the 1970s to the 50s for those born in the 1980s.[55,56] Families must manage their children and foster self-reliance, enabling them as adults to independently manage their daily intensive treatment regimen. The cystic fibrosis treatment burden is significant; health care expenditures for cystic fibrosis are 22 times higher than for the general population.[57]

Several studies have reported analyses using the Cystic Fibrosis Foundation (CFF) Patient Registry data. Researchers found that mortality and morbidity rates for individuals with cystic fibrosis were higher for those who had public insurance than for those with private insurance coverage.[58] The health outcomes of pulmonary function and growth were worse for those enrolled in public insurance plans; those with public insurance had a three times greater mortality risk. Data from the cystic fibrosis patient registry showed that individuals with cystic fibrosis of lower socioeconomic status were at higher risk for decreased lung functioning and lower body mass index.[5] Schechter and colleagues[58] concluded that low socioeconomic status was a proxy for several environmental risks that adversely affect health status, and that access to care was not a factor.[58]

Individuals with cystic fibrosis of Hispanic descent were found to be at increased risk for higher rates of liver complications and worse lung functioning. Researchers concluded that the high rate of Hispanic mothers with less than a high school education may contribute to lower rates of adherence, because these women may not fully understand cystic fibrosis management responsibilities.[59]

Adult outcomes have been examined using the CFF patient registry. These data showed that 8% of individuals reported having less than a high school diploma, 26% graduated from high school, and 32% were college graduates.[5] Unemployment rates of adults with cystic fibrosis were 36%, and only 7% reported full-time employment.[5,60]

According to data from the CFF patient registry, 40.1% of patients were married or living together and 54.8% were single.[5] In 2008, 240 women with cystic fibrosis reported they were pregnant. Nearly 20% of adults with cystic fibrosis reported symptoms of depression.

The CFF, whose mission is "...to assure the development of the means to cure and control cystic fibrosis and to improve the quality of life for those with the disease," provides the leadership to achieve this mission.[5] Important functions of the CFF are to fund and accredit the 115 cystic fibrosis care centers nationwide: 95 care centers for adults and 50 affiliate programs. The CFF provides research support to researchers to advance the science to improve care outcomes for individuals with cystic fibrosis. Since 1982, the CFF has maintained the national CFF patient registry, which is the repository of data collected from more than 25,500 individuals with cystic fibrosis who receive services through the network of cystic fibrosis care centers. The ethnic profile of individuals in the CFF patient registry is as follows: white, 92%; Hispanic, 7.2%; and African American, 4.3%. Registry data compiled include demographic, diagnostic profile, and health use information. According to the 2008 patient registry report, approximately 46% of individuals enrolled in the database are 18 years and older, reflecting the improving survival rates.[5]

CFF has mandated that adult programs be established at cystic fibrosis care centers with patient populations that include 40 or more adults older than 18 years.[5] This program organization is referred to as the *1 center, 2 programs* model. Since 2000, pediatric programs have been expected to transfer patients to adult programs for care, with chronologic age as the primary criterion used for transfer. The guidance beyond this transfer requirement is less clear regarding health care transition planning. Only 18% of programs reported self-management training for youth. Fewer than 10% of cystic fibrosis care centers reported the criterion of achievement of self-management practice/skills as a component of the transition planning. Additionally, no clear guidance regarding psychosocial support has been established. Data on health care transition planning outcomes are limited, as is evidence supporting that the perceived satisfaction with transition planning resulted in positive/stable health outcomes. Clinical guidelines and clear and consistent definitions regarding practices related to health care transition planning will advance the progress toward attaining the evidence needed.[61]

Comprehensive health care transition planning for young adults with cystic fibrosis is limited because typical peer support programs are not possible due to the threat of cross-infection among cystic fibrosis survivors. This lack of face-to-face contact among peers unfortunately prevents opportunities to talk, meet, and share information.[61] This constraint regarding live peer support has resulted in the development of electronic alternatives, such as online groups, wherein individuals with cystic fibrosis are able to meet each other and access online transition resources. The peer support Web site can be accessed at www.portCF.org.

NATIONAL EFFORTS

Various organized efforts have been undertaken to gather data on the long-term outcomes of emerging adults and older who are childhood cancer survivors or have cystic fibrosis or congenital heart disease. Data gathered on those with spina bifida have been described in other articles elsewhere in this issue. The most comprehensive efforts have been implemented by the consortium of 26 pediatric cancer centers in the United States and Canada that provide services to children and adolescents diagnosed with cancer.[40] Efforts to establish the CCSS consortium to collect data on childhood cancer survivors began in 1990. The data collection efforts have been extensive, involving surveys and specimen collections beginning in the mid-1990s to the present. The CCSS data set has provided investigators with a resource to examine a wide variety of topics pertaining to survivorship, ranging from psychosocial issues and health system use to morbidity and mortality issues. More than a 100 publications on survivorship topics have been generated from analyses of the CCSS data set.[40]

The CFF patient registry, although less ambitious in scope, also has been a valuable data set resource for cystic fibrosis researchers. Data collected includes information about height, weight, genotype, pulmonary function, pancreatic enzyme use, hospitalizations, home management, and complications related to cystic fibrosis. Selected data on adult outcomes are available, including pregnancies, employment, level of education, and marital status.[5]

The Centers for Disease Control and Prevention is currently funding efforts to establish a national patient registry for children and youth with spina bifida from birth to 21 years. Initially, demographic, diagnostic, and health care use data were collected, and efforts are underway to expand the range of data collected to include psychosocial and developmental items.

Recommendations have been made to create a national registry to track adults with CHD to better understand their biopsychosocial long-term outcomes. Currently, data collected on transitioning youth and adults with CHD in the United States have been limited to clusters or larger centers that treat adults with CHD. In Canada, several cohort studies have been conducted, with some of these findings cited previously; however, these efforts require more funding support to be sustained.

Establishment of national registries to track the outcomes of adults according to diagnostic classifications is needed to track and monitor long-term biopsychosocial outcomes. Other methods of longitudinal data collection (eg, Web sites, tracking systems, publicly available administrative data sets) must be considered to capture the lived experience for youth and families who cannot or decline to be enrolled in registries. Through these efforts, evidence will be gathered to better inform stakeholders about the need for treatment modalities to prevent, ameliorate, and eliminate late effects, complications, secondary conditions, and illnesses. Additionally, data on the indicators of successful adaptation to adulthood can be gathered as a means to inform on the status of adults with childhood-acquired chronic conditions compared with the general population. Outcomes data will provide information on the design of health care transition planning services needed, whether it involves additional screening, intervention programs, or support services.

SUMMARY

National and regional efforts have been undertaken to improve adult outcomes through the development of new systems and services to facilitate the healthy transition and transfer of patients with chronic conditions to adult health care services and ensure successful adult adaptation. Considerable emphasis has been placed on improving the delivery of medical care as the primary method of improving adult outcomes. In contrast, the efforts to develop a new online spina bifida resource, based on the Life Course Model and useful for a broad range of stakeholders—professionals and consumers alike—has focused on the family's and child's development of self-management competencies. This approach is unique when contrasted with the other efforts described, because it is focused on consumer skill-building based on the belief that effective self-management can be an important way to prevent complications and illnesses, minimize the emergence of secondary conditions, and foster successful adaptation to adulthood. It is also grounded in the principles of normal child development and the International Classification of Functioning, Disability and Health (ICF). The ICF has attained global recognition as a framework for describing positive, functional outcomes for individuals with chronic conditions.

REFERENCES

1. Reiss J, Gibson R. Health care transition: destinations unknown. Pediatrics 2002; 110(6 Pt 2):1307–14.
2. American Academy of Pediatrics AAoFP, American College of Physicians-American Society of Internal Medicine. A consensus statement on health care transitions for young adults with special health care needs. Pediatrics 2002;110(6 Pt 2):1304–6.
3. Betz CL. Transition of adolescents with special health care needs: review and analysis of the literature. Issues Compr Pediatr Nurs 2004;27:179–240.
4. Binks JA, Barden WS, Burke TA, et al. What do we really know about the transition to adult-centered health care? A focus on cerebral palsy and spina bifida. Arch Phys Med Rehabil 2007;88(8):1064–73.
5. Cystic Fibrosis Foundation. Patient registry: annual data report 2008. Available at: http://www.cff.org/UploadedFiles/research/ClinicalResearch/2008-Patient-Registry-Report.pdf. Accessed July 27, 2010.
6. Anie KA, Telfair J, Sickle Cell Disease Transition Study Working Group. Multi-site study of transition in adolescents with sickle cell disease in the United Kingdom and the United States. Int J Adolesc Med Health 2005;17(2):169–78.
7. Telfair J, Alleman-Velez PL, Dickens P, et al. Quality health care for adolescents with special health-care needs: issues and clinical implications. J Pediatr Nurs 2005;20(1):15–24.
8. Adult Congenital Heart Association. Available at: http://www.achaheart.org/index.php. Accessed July 27, 2010.
9. Bowman RM, McLone DG, Grant JA, et al. Spina bifida outcome: a 25-year prospective. Pediatr Neurosurg 2001;34(3):114–20.
10. Report of the British Cardiac Society Working Party. Grown-up congenital heart (GUCH) disease: current needs and provision of service for adolescents and adults with congenital heart disease in the UK. Heart 2002;88(Suppl 1):i1–14.
11. Moons P, Van Deyk K, Dedroog D, et al. Prevalence of cardiovascular risk factors in adults with congenital heart disease. Eur J Cardiovasc Prev Rehabil 2006; 13(4):612–6.
12. Marelli AJ, Mackie AS, Ionescu-Ittu R, et al. Congenital heart disease in the general population: changing prevalence and age distribution. Circulation 2007;115(2):163–72.
13. Hoffman JIE, Kaplan S, Liberthson RR. Prevalence of congenital heart disease. Am Heart J 2004;147(3):425–39.
14. Marelli AJ, Therrien J, Mackie AS, et al. Planning the specialized care of adult congenital heart disease patients: from numbers to guidelines; an epidemiologic approach. Am Heart J 2009;157(1):1–8.
15. Niwa K, Perloff JK, Webb GD, et al. Survey of specialized tertiary care facilities for adults with congenital heart disease. Int J Cardiol 2004;96(2):211–6.
16. Moons P, Siebens K, De Geest S, et al. A pilot study of expenditures on, and utilization of resources in, health care in adults with congenital heart disease. Cardiol Young 2001;11(3):301–13.
17. Shirodaria CC, Gwilt DJ, Gatzoulis MA. Joint outpatient clinics for the adult with congenital heart disease at the district general hospital: an alternative model of care. Int J Cardiol 2005;103(1):47–50.
18. Webb G. Improving the care of Canadian adults with congenital heart disease. Can J Cardiol 2005;21(10):833–8.
19. Yeung E, Kay J, Roosevelt GE, et al. Lapse of care as a predictor for morbidity in adults with congenital heart disease. Int J Cardiol 2008;125(1):62–5.

20. Warnes CA, Liberthson R, Danielson GK, et al. Task force 1: the changing profile of congenital heart disease in adult life. J Am Coll Cardiol 2001;37(5):1170–5.

21. Warnes CA, Williams RG, Bashore TM, et al. ACC/AHA 2008 Guidelines for the Management of Adults With Congenital Heart Disease: Executive Summary: a report of the American College of Cardiology/American Heart Association Task Force on Practice Guidelines (Writing Committee to Develop Guidelines for the Management of Adults With Congenital Heart Disease): Developed in Collaboration With the American Society of Echocardiography, Heart Rhythm Society, International Society for Adult Congenital Heart Disease, Society for Cardiovascular Angiography and Interventions, and Society of Thoracic Surgeons. Circulation 2008;118(23):2395–451.

22. Webb GD, Williams RG. Care of the adult with congenital heart disease: introduction. J Am Coll Cardiol 2001;37(5):1166.

23. Child JS, Collins-Nakai RL, Alpert JS, et al. Task force 3: workforce description and educational requirements for the care of adults with congenital heart disease. J Am Coll Cardiol 2001;37(5):1183–7.

24. Foster E, Graham TP Jr, Driscoll DJ, et al. Task force 2: special health care needs of adults with congenital heart disease. J Am Coll Cardiol 2001;37(5):1176–83.

25. Landzberg MJ, Murphy DJ Jr, Davidson WR Jr, et al. Task force 4: organization of delivery systems for adults with congenital heart disease. J Am Coll Cardiol 2001; 37(5):1187–93.

26. Skorton DJ, Garson A Jr, Fox JM, et al. Task force 5: adults with congenital heart disease: access to care. J Am Coll Cardiol 2001;37(5):1193–8.

27. Ries LAG, Eisner MP, Kosary CL, et al. SEER cancer statistics review: 1973–1998. Bethesda (MD): National Cancer Institute; 2001.

28. Albritton K, Bleyer WA. The management of cancer in the older adolescent. Eur J Cancer 2003;39(18):2584–99.

29. Blaauwbroek R, Tuinier W, Meyboom-de Jong B, et al. Shared care by paediatric oncologists and family doctors for long-term follow-up of adult childhood cancer survivors: a pilot study. Lancet Oncol 2008;9(3):232–8.

30. Jemal A, Siegel R, Ward E, et al. Cancer statistics, 2007. CA Cancer J Clin 2007; 57(1):43–66.

31. Hewitt W, Weinter SL, Simone JV, editors. Childhood cancer survivorship: improving care and quality of life. Washington, DC: National Academies Press; 2003.

32. Boman KK, Lindblad F, Hjern A. Long-term outcomes of childhood cancer survivors in Sweden: a population-based study of education, employment, and income. Cancer 2010;116(5):1385–91.

33. Yeh JM, Nekhlyudov L, Goldie SJ, et al. A model-based estimate of cumulative excess mortality in survivors of childhood cancer. Ann Intern Med 2010;152(7): 409–17.

34. Bhatia S, Constine LS. Late morbidity after successful treatment of children with cancer. Cancer J 2009;15(3):174–80.

35. CureSearch: Children's Oncology Group. Long-term follow-up guidelines for survivors of childhood, adolescent, and young adult cancers. Available at: http://www.childrensoncologygroup.org/pdf/LTFUGuidelines.pdf. Accessed July 27, 2010.

36. Oeffinger KC, Nathan PC, Kremer LC. Challenges after curative treatment for childhood cancer and long-term follow up of survivors. Pediatr Clin North Am 2008;55(1):251–73.

37. Han JW, Kwon SY, Won SC, et al. Comprehensive clinical follow-up of late effects in childhood cancer survivors shows the need for early and well-timed intervention. Ann Oncol 2009;20(7):1170–7.

38. Oeffinger KC, Robison LL. Childhood cancer survivors, late effects, and a new model for understanding survivorship. JAMA 2007;297(24):2762–4.
39. Janson C, Leisenring W, Cox C, et al. Predictors of marriage and divorce in adult survivors of childhood cancers: a report from the Childhood Cancer Survivor Study. Cancer Epidemiol Biomarkers Prev 2009;18(10):2626–35.
40. Robison LL, Armstrong GT, Boice JD, et al. The Childhood Cancer Survivor Study: a National Cancer Institute-supported resource for outcome and intervention research. J Clin Oncol 2009;27(14):2308–18.
41. Schultz KA, Ness KK, Whitton J, et al. Behavioral and social outcomes in adolescent survivors of childhood cancer: a report from the childhood cancer survivor study. J Clin Oncol 2007;25(24):3649–56.
42. Servitzoglou M, Papadatou D, Tsiantis I, et al. Psychosocial functioning of young adolescent and adult survivors of childhood cancer. Support Care Cancer 2008;16(1):29–36.
43. McDougall J, Tsonis M. Quality of life in survivors of childhood cancer: a systematic review of the literature (2001–2008). Support Care Cancer 2009;17(10):1231–46.
44. Meeske KA, Patel SK, Palmer SN, et al. Factors associated with health-related quality of life in pediatric cancer survivors. Pediatr Blood Cancer 2007;49(3):298–305.
45. Gurney JG, Krull KR, Kadan-Lottick N, et al. Social outcomes in the Childhood Cancer Survivor Study cohort. J Clin Oncol 2009;27(14):2390–5.
46. Crom DB, Lensing SY, Rai SN, et al. Marriage, employment, and health insurance in adult survivors of childhood cancer. J Cancer Surviv 2007;1(3):237–45.
47. Thompson AL, Marsland AL, Marshal MP, et al. Romantic relationships of emerging adult survivors of childhood cancer. Psychooncology 2009;18(7):767–74.
48. Klosky JL, Cash DK, Buscemi J, et al. Factors influencing long-term follow-up clinic attendance among survivors of childhood cancer. J Cancer Surviv 2008;2(4):225–32.
49. Oeffinger KC, Wallace WH. Barriers to follow-up care of survivors in the United States and the United Kingdom. Pediatr Blood Cancer 2006;46(2):135–42.
50. Clarke SA, Eiser C. Health behaviours in childhood cancer survivors: a systematic review. Eur J Cancer 2007;43(9):1373–84.
51. Knijnenburg SL, Kremer LC, van den Bos C, et al. Health information needs of childhood cancer survivors and their family. Pediatr Blood Cancer 2010;54(1):123–7.
52. Britton LJ, Thrasher S, Gutierrez H. Creating a culture of improvement: experience of a pediatric cystic fibrosis center. J Nurs Care Qual 2008;23(2):115–20 [quiz: 121–2].
53. Lai HJ, Cheng Y, Cho H, et al. Association between initial disease presentation, lung disease outcomes, and survival in patients with cystic fibrosis. Am J Epidemiol 2004;159(6):537–46.
54. Kulich M, Rosenfeld M, Goss CH, et al. Improved survival among young patients with cystic fibrosis. J Pediatr 2003;142(6):631–6.
55. Farrell PM, Rosenstein BJ, White TB, et al. Guidelines for diagnosis of cystic fibrosis in newborns through older adults: Cystic Fibrosis Foundation consensus report. J Pediatr 2008;153(2):S4–14.
56. Elborn JS, Shale DJ, Britton JR. Cystic fibrosis: current survival and population estimates to the year 2000. Thorax 1991;46(12):881–5 [Erratum appears in Thorax 1992;47(2):139].

57. Foundation CF. Patient registry, 2005 Annual data report to the center directors. Bethesda (MD): Cystic Fibrosis Foundation; 2005.

58. Schechter MS, Shelton BJ, Margolis PA, et al. The association of socioeconomic status with outcomes in cystic fibrosis patients in the United States. Am J Respir Crit Care Med 2001;163(6):1331–7.

59. Watts KD, Seshadri R, Sullivan C, et al. Increased prevalence of risk factors for morbidity and mortality in the US Hispanic CF population. Pediatr Pulmonol 2009;44(6):594–601.

60. Marelich GP, Cross CE. Cystic fibrosis in adults. From researcher to practitioner. West J Med 1996;164(4):321–34.

61. Tuchman LK, Slap GB, Britto MT. Transition to adult care. experiences and expectations of adolescents with a chronic illness. Child Care Health Dev 2008;34(5): 557–63.

Urinary Continence across the Life Course

Kathryn Smith, RN, MN[a,b,*], Stacey Mizokawa, PhD[a],
Ann Neville-Jan, PhD, OTR/L[c], Kristy Macias[a]

KEYWORDS

- Spina bifida • Continence • Urologic care • Quality of life

Spina bifida is the most common defect of the central nervous system, affecting approximately 1000 newborns each year in the United States.[1,2] The Centers for Disease Control and Prevention (CDC) estimates that as many as 166,000 individuals with spina bifida live in the United States.[3] Spina bifida is a congenital malformation of the spine with abnormal neural tube closure occurring between the third and fourth weeks of gestation, and most frequently affecting the lumbar and sacral regions.[4] Liptak and El Samra[2] characterize it as the most complex birth defect compatible with survival. Most children with spina bifida have a normal urinary tract at birth,[5] although renal damage and renal failure are among the most severe complications of spina bifida,[6,7] resulting from lack of appropriate innervation of the bladder, and the effects of the neurogenic bladder on the kidneys.[5] Thirty to forty percent of individuals with spina bifida exhibit varying degrees of renal dysfunction throughout life,[8] and renal failure is the most common cause of death.[9] Before ventricular shunting, survival rates for children with spina bifida were low, and therefore "urologic intervention was rarely necessary."[4(p 72)] With improving technologies and clinical care, most patients can be expected to live into adulthood,[10] thus prevention of urologic complications, in particular renal failure, and promotion of continence have become critical.

This article reviews the literature regarding urinary continence, and discusses issues across the lifespan and implications for clinical practice. The pediatrician's role in the urologic care of children with spina bifida focuses on serving as the medical home for the child, assisting the child and family to become independent in care, promoting urinary continence, and monitoring for the development of urologic complications

[a] Department of Pediatrics, University of Southern California (USC), University Center for Excellence in Developmental Disabilities (UCEDD), Childrens Hospital Los Angeles (CHLA), 4650 Sunset Boulevard, MS #53 Los Angeles, CA 90027, USA
[b] Department of Pediatrics, Keck School of Medicine-USC, 1975 Zonal Avenue, Los Angeles, CA 90089, USA
[c] Department of Occupational Science & Occupational Therapy, University of Southern California, 1540 Alcazar Street, CHP-133, Los Angeles, CA 90089, USA
* Corresponding author. Department of Pediatrics, University of Southern California (USC), University Center for Excellence in Developmental Disabilities (UCEDD), Childrens Hospital Los Angeles (CHLA), 4650 Sunset Boulevard, MS #53 Los Angeles, CA 90027.
E-mail address: kasmith@chla.usc.edu

Pediatr Clin N Am 57 (2010) 997–1011
doi:10.1016/j.pcl.2010.07.018
0031-3955/10/$ – see front matter © 2010 Published by Elsevier Inc.

that threaten the health of the kidneys, in collaboration with the spina bifida special care center and other specialists. In addition, the medical home coordinates care with providers and services in the community, and works with the child and family as they transition to adult care.

GOALS OF UROLOGIC CARE

More than 90% of children with spina bifida have normal upper tracts at birth,[5,7] although, if unattended, 50% will experience deterioration.[7] There are 4 goals of urologic care for the individual with spina bifida: (1) prevention of urinary tract infection, (2) preservation of renal function to avoid chronic renal failure and end-stage renal disease, (3) prevention of decubitus ulcers through promotion of continence, and (4) facilitation of urinary continence and independence in bladder care. Achievement of these goals is assumed to enable meaningful participation in activities (including adult sexual experiences, and typical vocations and avocations), promote positive self-esteem, and improve quality of life.[5,6,11] Successful therapeutic interventions require a working knowledge of the pathophysiology, effective treatments, normal developmental processes, and effective means of empowering parents and children to master urinary continence as a means to promote health and greatly improve activity and participation in typical societal roles as adults.

Urinary continence is a significant factor in estimating the quality of life for children with spina bifida and their families. Percentages of children who are continent range from 78% to 90%.[4,7,12] Children with spina bifida are at risk for symptoms of depression and anxiety, as well as lower levels of self-concept compared with their nonaffected peers.[13,14] This may be because of teasing, feeling self-conscious about their bodies and physical appearance, and social isolation. Daily bladder management can become burdensome for parents and children, and, as children struggle with negative feelings, parents may experience frustration with their child's bladder and bowel management programs, or adherence to these programs, resulting in tension between parents, children, and team members. Previous research conducted with other chronic conditions suggests that family cohesion is related to better treatment adherence,[15] whereas family conflict has been associated with poorer treatment adherence.[16] Siblings may also experience frustration with their brother's or sister's bladder or bowel management programs, especially if they attend the same school or share mutual friends. We have heard siblings complain about being embarrassed about catheters being left in the bathroom, where friends may discover them. However, the research on the adjustment of siblings of spina bifida patients has been mixed, and not focused on the effect of incontinence on siblings' emotional functioning.[17] Nevertheless, because spina bifida care affects the entire family, it is important to overall family functioning and quality of life to identify the factors that promote successful bladder and bowel continence programs for children who have spina bifida.

MANAGEMENT OF THE NEUROGENIC BLADDER

In addition to causing incontinence that may affect social functioning, a neurogenic bladder can cause damage to the entire urinary tract, including the kidneys. Thirty percent of the deaths in adult patients with spina bifida can be attributed to the urinary tract.[18,19] Attainment of urinary and bowel continence is a critical component of the overall management strategy for neurogenic bladder, especially now that most children with spina bifida can expect to live into adulthood. Furthermore, because abnormal bladder function has been shown to be the principal cause of renal damage,[20] the protection of upper urinary tract and management of continence issues often go hand in hand.

Studies for evaluation and monitoring of the urinary tract include regular renal and bladder ultrasonography, voiding cystourethrography, and urodynamics testing to provide baseline information, help detect early changes, identify children at high risk for kidney damage or poor bladder function, and assisting to identify a management plan.[6,20–24] The voiding cystourethrogram can rule out vesicoureteral reflux and assess the bladder outlet.[24] The urodynamics study is a functional evaluation of the bladder and the urethra and provides information related to bladder capacity, compliance, leak pressure, overactive bladder contractions, bladder areflexia, and bladder sphincter synergy and dyssynergy. Typically, patients are followed conservatively when studies are normal, being yearly at least through ages 3 to 4 years[5] and continuing through adulthood, because renal function may deteriorate.[7]

Medical Management

General treatment strategies for urologic care for the child with spina bifida include pharmacotherapy and regular bladder emptying through clean, intermittent catheterization (CIC). During the newborn period, renal and bladder ultrasound is typically performed within 48 hours of birth to assess the urinary tract and postvoid residual, and allow for the provision of prophylactic antibiotics if hydronephrosis is present. If the infant retains a significant amount of urine, or is unable to void spontaneously, scheduled CIC is performed, adjusted based on the volume of residual urine. A wet diaper does not imply normal voiding, because it may represent overflow incontinence, and a low-pressure bladder must be maintained from birth to prevent kidney damage.[6] Further baseline studies including a voiding cystourethrogram and urodynamic evaluation are performed several months after closure of the spinal defect to determine whether the bladder is functioning properly.[5,6,24]

Two general approaches exist for the management of the urinary tract in the newborn period: an early preventive/anticipatory intervention (proactive) management approach and a wait and see (reactive) approach.[24] In the proactive approach, the infant at risk for upper urinary tract deterioration is identified and treatment is initiated before problems are evident. In the retrospective or reactive approach, the infant is followed closely and treatment is initiated at the first sign of problems. Good results exist with both approaches but large, multisite studies are needed to determine the most effective approach. About 25% of newborns leave the hospital having CIC performed by the parents.[5] In infants who do not respond to CIC and medications, vesicostomy is a safe and effective alternative.[5]

Medical therapy includes CIC and anticholinergic therapy to adequately empty the bladder and protect the upper tract.[25] Asymptomatic bacteremia is common and does not require treatment in most cases.[5] Symptomatic infection occurs less than 30% of the time, with asymptomatic bacteremia present in more than 70% of cases.[26,27] Indications for treatment of urinary tract infection include pain with catheterization, gross hematuria, worsening incontinence, and abdominal discomfort. Because fever is a less-specific indicator in children, it should not be used alone. Odor and cloudy urine without other signs of possible infection should be treated with increased hydration.[24] Prevention of the development of resistant infection is important, and thus antibiotic treatment should only be used when clearly indicated.

The use of CIC with or without anticholinergic medications such as oxybutinin permits low-pressure storage and complete bladder emptying, factors that are considered essential for maintenance of upper and lower urinary tract health. Since the introduction of CIC by Lapides and colleagues[28] in 1972, significant advances have been made in the management of children with neurogenic bladder, but CIC remains the most popular option to achieve continence and prevent upper urinary tract deterioration.[7]

Surgical Management

Some children may require urinary tract reconstruction to prevent deterioration of the urinary tract such as bladder augmentation, urethral continence surgery, and continent urinary diversion.[25,29–32] About 50% of children with spina bifida may eventually require some form of urologic surgery.[33] Indications for surgery include failure of medical management to produce a safe, low-pressure bladder, and deterioration of the upper urinary tract.[34] Surgery focuses on improving bladder capacity, lowering bladder pressure, and protecting upper tracts from damage,[7] and is generally reserved for persistent incontinence,[5] to aid in catheterization via catheterizable channels, and to prevent further damage to the kidneys. With difficulties catheterizing the urethra because of excess weight, or difficulty reaching or seeing the area, continent catheterizable channels can aid in achievement of continence. However, risks include stomal stenosis and leakage, and it requires a lifelong commitment to catheterization.[5] For those adults who have had bladder augmentation, long-term follow-up for development of malignancies is needed and typically consists of cystoscopy beginning 10 years after the initial procedure.[35]

Surgeries to increase resistance of the bladder outlet, including injection of bulking agents, bladder neck reconstruction, and placement of bladder slings and artificial urinary sphincters can be performed, although they are not all successful. Bladder neck closure with creation of a continent catheterizable conduit may be needed if all else fails, and bladder augmentation is often performed at the same time. Bladder neck closure is effective for achieving continence but success depends on compliance with CIC. However, according to Nguyen and Baskin,[36] 85% of patients ultimately achieved urinary continence 2 years after surgery. There is an increased risk for stomal stenosis and bladder stones, incontinence, and infection.[5,6,25,36,37] Complications from bladder augmentation can include metabolic imbalance, stone formation, chronic urinary tract infection, bladder rupture, and tumors.[5]

During childhood, toilet training and continence become primary goals.[5,24] Surveillance of the urinary tract for bladder hostility or deterioration of the upper tract continues.[25] Children can begin to learn self-catheterization during the early school years.[25] Before this time, parents can narrate the catheterization procedure while they are performing it, and have children help with activities such as opening packages, or putting away supplies, to begin to engage them in the process. Optimally, the child should move toward independence in bladder care during the school years whenever possible.

For adolescents, facilitation of urinary continence and preservation of renal function continue to be primary goals. Clayton reports that continence can be achieved in as many as 90% of patients.[25] Adolescence is an important time to solidify self-care skills and ensure a complete understanding of the condition to prepare for independent living, postsecondary education, romantic relationships, and gainful employment.[5] The risk of renal damage and hypertension increases with age, so close monitoring with follow-up into and through adulthood is needed.[7,24]

Any deterioration in urinary function must be examined, because one of the most common causes is tethered cord,[4,5] which occurs in 15% to 25% of patients, commonly presenting between 2 and 8 years of age. It is caused by adhesions between the spinal cord and the repaired dura mater, with resultant ischemic changes from tension on the cord. There is the potential for improvement after cord release,[11] so early attention to symptoms is important.

Despite advances in care, urinary incontinence, urinary tract infections, and threats to renal health remain significant problems for children and adults with spina bifida. Few prospective studies have evaluated the efficacy and safety of therapies that are currently used, and significant variation in care exists from region to region, and practitioner to practitioner. A urologic standard of care for children with spina bifida is yet to be established because few data are available to adequately evaluate currently available therapies.

Outcomes of Treatment

The effectiveness of existing therapies should be evaluated not only on their medical outcomes but also on their effects on the quality of life of the patients and their families. In our recent work, the relationship between quality of life and continence regimens has been inconsistent, possibly because measuring quality of life in a child with spina bifida is difficult. One reason why quality of life in children with spina bifida has been hard to measure is because there are few tools to assess it. Although there has been debate about whether general health-related quality of life (HRQoL) should be assessed, or whether it is preferable to obtain disease-specific measures of quality of life, for assessing changes related to treatment, disease-specific measures are preferred.[38] One HRQoL instrument for spina bifida has been developed,[39] but, in a review of quality-of-life measures, some shortcomings were identified.[40] However, it is the only spina bifida–specific measure of quality of life in children published and available at the present time. In addition, no information about the quality of life for children with spina bifida has included the use of qualitative methods such as interviews or focus groups.

Another limitation of previous research in quality of life is the reliance on parents and providers to rate quality. Although it is difficult to collect this type of information for very young children, it is thought that children should rate their own quality of life whenever possible.[38] Previous studies have shown that the family's experience of their child's medical condition is not as negative as health care providers perceive it to be.[41] Thus, it is important to seek information about quality of life from the children directly and, if this is not possible, from their parents.

CONTINENCE FROM A DEVELOPMENTAL PERSPECTIVE
Young Children

Bladder incontinence in infants and toddlers may not be obvious to others because all children in this age group wear diapers, thus the focus of bladder programs for this age group is primarily on optimizing medical outcomes. During the preschool years, bladder incontinence becomes an issue that is recognized in school, in public, and by the child with spina bifida. Preschool children with spina bifida recognize the differences between themselves and their nonaffected peers[42] and begin to ask questions about why they urinate differently than their friends. It is important for parents to be prepared to answer such questions and openly discuss these matters with their children.

Some parents wonder whether they should attempt to toilet train their child with spina bifida, because most individuals with spina bifida have some degree of incontinence. Only about 15% of those with spina bifida achieve complete bladder and bowel continence without the use of medications and CIC.[43] For children with spina bifida, bowel and bladder control are typically achieved later than for their nonaffected peers

(6–8 years old), if at all. However, the expectation that the child will need to participate in their continence program and gradually manage it independently should be established early, around 2 or 3 years of age. Although children with spina bifida may not develop full continence, they should be encouraged to participate in their continence program as early as possible.[44] Children of this age are naturally curious about the bathroom and should be allowed to go into the bathroom[43] as well as participate in the continence program in developmentally appropriate ways. For example, although a 2 year old is too young to insert a catheter without assistance, they can be responsible for getting the catheter and giving it to their parent. Or, the child may wash their hands before and after catheterization. It is also important to communicate the expectation that the child will learn to perform CIC independently. A parent or caregiver may convey this intention by talking through the steps of CIC and having the child watch how it is done (instead of lying on their back passively), even before the child is ready to learn how to insert the catheter. Setting the stage for being independent in self-care during the early childhood years is essential if independence is to be achieved during the elementary school years.

School-age Children

By the time a child with spina bifida is in elementary school, the parents should be considering ways of increasing their child's independence in managing the continence program. The guidelines for spina bifida care published by the Spina Bifida Association[45] indicate that children should be taught self-catheterization when they are school aged (6–11 years old). It is generally accepted that, by the beginning of middle school, children should be fully independent in self-catheterization and should ideally have achieved urinary continence.

As they mature, achieving continence becomes increasingly important to children with spina bifida. It is during the school years that increases in teasing and exclusion are typically seen, and issues with low self-esteem related to incontinence begin to emerge. Moore and colleagues[46] asked spina bifida patients 7 to 19 years old to rate their academic, social, and athletic competence, as well as their physical appearance, behavior, and self-worth. The data were analyzed by continence status, gender, and other variables. In general, the findings revealed no significant differences between patients who were continent (ie, did not use protective undergarments) and the control group. However, those who were incontinent rated themselves lower in social acceptance and global self-concept than the control group. Gender differences also emerged: girls who were continent rated themselves higher in social acceptance and self-worth than girls who were incontinent; boys who were continent rated themselves higher in scholastic competence, social acceptance, appearance, and behavior compared with their peers who were incontinent.[46] The sample contained too few patients to make additional comparisons by age.

The development of good social skills becomes especially important during the school years. People with good social skills are able to make more friends, thus increasing their support systems, and have a better sense of how appropriately to share information about their medical condition with others, how much information to share, with whom to share it, and how to deal with questions or teasing that is likely to arise. By developing good social skills, a child with spina bifida can also ensure greater participation in developmentally and age-appropriate activities, such as having play dates, going to birthday parties, and going to sleepovers. Establishing such social activities at this age increases the likelihood that participation in age-appropriate activities will continue into adolescence.

During these years, it is also important to explain the concepts of appropriate and inappropriate touches, who is allowed to touch their bodies, and what to do if someone tries to touch them inappropriately. Because many children with spina bifida have decreased sensation in their genitals, and because so many caregivers (eg, parents, physicians, nurses) examine these parts of their bodies routinely, they may not perceive the same ownership of these parts as nonaffected peers. Thus, there may have to be additional teaching about what inappropriate touches are and how to recognize them. However, because children with disabilities are at increased risk of being sexually abused,[47] and because children with spina bifida often require assistance in their bladder care from others, it is important to review this information with children in a calm, matter-of-fact, nonthreatening manner.

Adolescents

Ideally, adolescents with spina bifida are independent in their continence programs. If they are not, it is hoped that they are motivated to become independent because they desire the freedom to participate in typical adolescent activities like playing sports, going out with their friends, or spending the night away from home. This is more likely if developing age-appropriate social skills is a focus of their school years.

Several studies have alerted health care practitioners to important medical and social needs of adolescents and young adults with spina bifida and their families.[48–51] One recent descriptive study[52] found that, although adolescents with spina bifida had generally positive attitudes and were independent in self-care, they were not participating in the full range of adolescent activities. This finding leads to questions about the role of bowel and bladder incontinence in this lack of social participation. Another study found that adolescents and their parents had significantly divergent perspectives about the needs of the adolescent.[53] How does this extend to issues of incontinence and what are the perceptions of practitioners to the needs of children with spina bifida? Although studies are beginning to explain the overall attitudes and beliefs of individuals with spina bifida, they have not examined the complex subjective experience of living with spina bifida while managing the problems related to incontinence.

Research has shown that the transfer of responsibility for catheterization transitions from parent to child gradually over time, beginning in middle childhood.[54] Although expecting a child to self-catheterize before they are ready may have negative consequences (as seen in children with other chronic conditions[55]), not allowing a child to assume this responsibility when they are ready and capable of doing so may also thwart the transition to independence.[54] Stepansky and colleagues[54] suggest that, because parents of children with spina bifida tend to be overprotective[56], adolescents with spina bifida may be more dependent on their parents than is necessary. Their longitudinal research suggests that, as children get older, conflicts related to medical issues are related to decreased medical adherence.[54] Therefore, more information about how to assess readiness for this transition, as well as how to assist parents in transferring the responsibilities to their children, needs to be researched.

Adolescence is a difficult time in general, but being an adolescent with spina bifida is especially challenging. In addition to the typical issues of adolescence, a teenager with spina bifida must contend with managing their continence program while out with friends or in the context of dating (and possibly sexual) relationships. For these reasons, the Spina Bifida Association guidelines for spina bifida care suggest that teaching about intimacy, sexuality, and sexual functioning are key urological interventions for this age group.[45]

Adolescents with spina bifida may also rebel in ways that could ultimately cause themselves harm. Not only could refusing to do CIC affect the adolescent's physical health, it could affect them socially if bladder or bowel accidents occur as a result, or if odors become obvious. Although such rebellion is considered typical and developmentally appropriate, it nevertheless must be addressed to prevent long-term health and psychological consequences.

Adulthood

Medical advancements, such as the development of the shunt and urological surgeries, have greatly improved the survival rate of infants born with spina bifida. The literature suggests that children born with spina bifida who receive proper medical care and support for incorporating wellness interventions into their lifestyles can have a normal life expectancy. However, there are few reports describing outcomes into later adulthood, making it difficult to determine life expectancy.[57] Continuing challenges facing adults with spina bifida and their health care providers are urinary incontinence and potential kidney damage. Renal failure is the most frequently reported cause of death in adults with spina bifida,[7,19] and kidney infection is a frequent cause for hospital admissions.[58] In a study of urinary and fecal incontinence among young adults in the Netherlands,[59] researchers found that, of the 179 patients studied, 63% used diapers. Diapers were used more often for urinary incontinence (90.7% of those who used diapers). Moreover, adults who wear diapers are susceptible to pressure ulcers as an additional serious medical complication.

Incontinence has repercussions for social participation. Incontinence at any age can be the source of embarrassment and humiliation. However, quantitative studies of adult quality of life have not shown a relationship between standard measures of quality of life and continence. Lemelle and colleagues[60] conducted a cross-sectional study of 460 patients, of whom 300 were adults, across 6 spina bifida centers in France. Using the Short Form (SF)-36 Health Survey to measure HRQoL, they found no relationship between HRQoL and continence. Surgical management and 2 domains of the SF-31 (without diversion and role physical; with continent diversion and general health) were significantly related. The investigators speculated that surgical management may result in more physical independence and thus positively affect this area of HRQoL. Standard quality of life measures may not adequately evaluate the effect of incontinence. In a study of young adults with spina bifida, Verhoef and colleagues[59] asked research participants whether they perceived incontinence (defined as an accident once a month or more) as a problem. They found that 69.7% (76) of patients who were incontinent (109) perceived it as a problem. Simply asking a question about the effect of incontinence on day-to-day life may result in more useful information about adult experiences and concerns.

Neville-Jan,[61] a woman with spina bifida, used a qualitative research methodology called autoethnography to describe her experiences growing up with spina bifida. Her account provides support for the positive effect of surgical urological intervention and the stigmatizing nature of incontinence. She states:

> Bladder incontinence became the most stigmatizing impairment for me. In 1970, I had a surgical procedure called an ileal conduit, which diverted urine from my bladder to an outside appliance on my abdomen. After the surgery I finally achieved independence. The following year, I left home, bound for New York City to study occupational therapy (61; p. 530).

Mobility impairments and incontinence intersect in different ways across adulthood. As ambulatory young adults age, they may be more susceptible to falls. Falls sometimes occur when rushing to go to the bathroom to avoid an accident.[62] Older adults who are wheelchair users may face similar challenges when bathrooms are not accessible and timing is a factor.

Urinary incontinence directly affects social participation. Sexuality and partnering are important areas of life in which adults with spina bifida who are incontinent may face restrictions. Several studies have identified that young adults who are incontinent tend to have limited sexual activity. Cardenas and colleagues[63] studied 121 adolescents and young adults between 15 and 35 years of age and found that those incontinent of urine were not likely to engage in sexual activity. Gatti and colleagues[64] studied the predictors of having a relationship and sexual activity in 290 patients with spina bifida. Patients ranged in age from 18 to 32 years, with a mean of age of 23.4 years. Urinary continence was a significant predictor of sexual partnering. Culleres and colleagues[65] conducted a prospective study of 143 adults with spina bifida to assess the effect of incontinence on sexual activity. They found that only 39% of the adults were active sexually. Most of these adults had lesions at lower levels, had a partner, and were working. Dicianno and colleagues[57] conducted a comprehensive review of the literature on spina bifida during the past 20 years. They reported that male and female adults with spina bifida who were incontinent were not likely to be sexually active. Medical providers should be alert to these issues and refer patients to the appropriate resources for help with both sexuality and incontinence.

We did not locate any studies that directly examined other areas of social participation, particularly employment, as it relates to incontinence in adults with spina bifida. However, the literature does suggest that individuals with spina bifida are limited in social participation. Buffart and colleagues[66] studied lifestyle factors in 51 adolescents and young adults with spina bifida (mean age of 21 years). More than half of the participants had problems related to social role functioning, particularly recreation and employment. Hunt and Oakeshott[67] followed a cohort of 54 individuals with spina bifida who survived to an average age of 35 years, and conducted a phone survey to access community living. Of the 54 survivors, 11 were continent, 13 were employed, and 11 drove cars at the time of the survey. The investigators did not report whether those who were incontinent had the most difficulty in social role performance but this is likely given the stigma associated with incontinence.

Longitudinal studies need to be conducted to assess the urological needs of young adults as they age and the influence of incontinence on community participation. Also, more needs to be understood about older adults with spina bifida. Clinically, multidisciplinary clinics need to be established for adults to manage issues related not just to urological impairments but to social role functioning, such as sexuality, partnering, and employment.

CLINICAL IMPLICATIONS

Given the great variability in needs and outcomes of children and youths with spina bifida,[68] individualization of treatment approaches is necessary within the context of recognized standards of care. Active engagement of family members and, when appropriate, the child in decision making is important to establish a long-term partnership in care. In addition, information sharing and collaboration between the community-based medical home, special care centers, and specialists enhances care delivery and improves outcomes.

Spina bifida is a condition in which family members, adolescents, and adult patients are responsible for performing most of the care. Thus, a comprehensive educational program that provides an overview of the condition, as well as short- and long-term care, helps to achieve the best possible outcomes for the child. Ideally, this educational program should be introduced in the neonatal intensive care unit and then continued during the first and subsequent visits to the spina bifida clinic. It may be helpful to provide families with literature or resources available on the Internet for them to explore. If possible, parents can be given a resource binder that includes information about spina bifida as well as a system for tracking medical appointments and relevant health information that can then be shared among providers to enhance coordination of care.

Providers need to be aware that such education is not a static event, but a dynamic process. The information provided to the family may not be well retained, especially when it is given during stressful times, and it may therefore need to be repeated. Written material used in collaboration with oral explanations is especially valuable, allowing parents to review the information at a later time, in a less stressful environment. Although initially education will be focused on the parents, it should transition to include the child as early as the child seems to be interested and capable of understanding. As the child becomes older, explanations may need to be revisited and updated to correspond with the child's increasing level of maturity. Likewise, important concepts need to be repeated frequently to assure that understanding is complete.

Providers should monitor continence outcomes as well as the effect of the continence programs on the child's and family's quality of life. As issues arise, referring back to the educational information previously provided and reminding the family of the expectations of the child's participation in the continence program will be necessary. In addition, close monitoring and frequent conversation allows the bladder management plan to be revised as needed to better meet the child's and family's needs and goals. The expectation that the child with spina bifida will be managing their own continence regimen by the end of elementary school needs to be established early and could be appropriately introduced during toddlerhood, when questions about potty training are likely to occur. If CIC is appropriate it can be introduced at this time. The literature identifies that children as young as 2 years old[69] and with an IQ as low as 60[70] have been able to self-catheterize. If not completely independent, it is expected that children with spina bifida should be allowed and encouraged to participate in 1 or more components of their continence routines so that they may gradually take over their self-care needs.

The occupational therapist can assess the fine motor skills needed for self-catheterization and, in collaboration with the nurse, begin a teaching program that may involve videos and dolls for simulation. Although this task may seem straightforward, the topic of independence in self-care needs to be addressed in a culturally sensitive and relevant manner, because not all cultural groups value or expect independence, especially for a child with a chronic health condition. Because children spend much of their time in school, it is also important to establish collaboration with health care providers in the child's school environment. The school nurse can greatly assist by reinforcing catheterization techniques, helping the child to monitor the status of the skin, and assist in maintaining a schedule to work toward the goals of maintaining normal renal function, achieving continence, and promoting independence.[71] Working collaboratively with the school nurse can encourage and maintain optimal continence outcomes in a child with spina bifida.

Medical management of incontinence is most frequently directed by the urologist, but the primary care provider serves important roles in reinforcing and monitoring the plan of care, assessing for complications such as urinary tract infections and skin breakdown, and promoting independence in self-care. Within the context of typical developmental expectations, the community and family environment, and the health care needs of the child, the medical home provider is well positioned to coordinate the health care and serve as a primary resource to the family. Although mentioned earlier, asymptomatic bacteremia is considered the norm and does not need to be aggressively treated with antibiotics. Odor, cloudy urine, or other vague symptoms should be treated with increased hydration. Antibiotics are indicated only with symptomatic infection to reduce the possibility of resistant microorganisms.

For those children who need urological surgery, it is important that the parents and, when appropriate, the child have an understanding of the surgical undertaking and the care that will be required after surgery.[25] This is especially important for children less than 11 years old, because research has shown that children this young have difficulty understanding aspects of youth assent, such as the procedure or protocol.[72] In these cases, drawings and diagrams may help children and families understand complex procedures and provide rationale for surgeries. A psychologist may help the family to cope with the stress of the hospitalization, or repeated hospitalizations, and pain management following the surgery.

As discussed earlier, more and more individuals born with spina bifida are surviving into adulthood, but spina bifida care for adults is not as well defined as it is for the pediatric population. Ideally, a multidisciplinary team that functions as a one-stop clinic should follow adults to assess the complex challenges that occur throughout adulthood,[7] but only a few such centers exist. Practitioners who see adult patients with spina bifida should not simply assume that pediatric protocols can continue to be followed. Changes in mobility status or the onset of other health conditions may affect urological management strategies and it is essential that kidney function continues to be monitored. For these reasons, it is important that pediatric practitioners prepare children and their families for the transition to adult care providers early, during late childhood or early adolescence. It is imperative that practitioners begin addressing their questions to the teen and young adult with spina bifida, not just the parents, and begin establishing the expectation that the young person will need to take over monitoring their health and the need for appointments or follow-up care. Again, transition to adult care is not an event but an ongoing process that takes years to complete successfully.

Although there have been tremendous advances in care for individuals with spina bifida, incontinence and damage to the upper urinary tract continue to be significant areas of concern for patients, family members, and their physicians. Collaborations and shared goals between patients, families, and providers can help children with spina bifida become healthy and productive adults.

REFERENCES

1. Boulet SL, Gambrell D, Shin M, et al. Racial/ethnic differences in the birth prevalence of spina bifida - United States 1995–2005. MMWR Morb Mortal Wkly Rep 2009;57:1409–13.
2. Liptak G, El Samra A. Optimizing health care for children with spina bifida. Dev Disabil Res Rev 2010;16:66–75.
3. Liptak GS, editor. The future is now: first world congress on spina bifida research and care. Washington, DC: Centers for Disease Control; 2010.
4. Netto JMB, Bastos AN, Figueiredo AA, et al. Spinal dysraphism: a neurosurgical review for the urologist. Rev Urol 2009;11:71–81.
5. Joseph DB. Current approaches to the urologic care of children with spina bifida. Curr Urol Rep 2008;9:151–7.

6. De Jong TP, Chrzan R, Klijn AJ. Treatment of the neurogenic bladder in spina bifida. Pediatr Nephrol 2008;23:889–96.

7. Ahmad I, Granitsiotis P. Urological follow-up of adult spina bifida patients. Neurourol Urodyn 2007;26:978–80.

8. Muller T, Arbeiter K, Aufricht C. Renal function in meningomyelocele: risk factors, chronic renal failure, renal replacement therapy and transplantation. Curr Opin Urol 2002;12:479–84.

9. Woodhouse CR. Myelomeningocele in young adults. BJU Int 2005;95:223–30.

10. Bowman RM, McLone DG, Grant JA, et al. Spina bifida outcome: a 25-year prospective. Pediatr Neurosurg 2001;34:114–20.

11. Clayton DB, Brock JW 3rd, Joseph DB. Urological management of spina bifida. Dev Disabil Res Rev 2010;16:88–95.

12. Dik A, Klijn A, van Gool JD, et al. Early start to therapy preserves kidney function in spina bifida patients. Eur Urol 2006;49:908–13.

13. Holmbeck GN, Westhoven VC, Phillips WS, et al. A multimethod, multi-informant, and multidimensional perspective on psychosocial adjustment in preadolescents with spina bifida. J Consult Clin Psychol 2003;71:782–95.

14. Shields N, Taylor NF, Dodd KJ. Self-concept in children with spina bifida compared with typically developing children. Dev Med Child Neurol 2008;50:733–43.

15. La Greca AM, Bearman KJ. Adherence to pediatric treatment regimens. In: MC Roberts, editor. Handbook of pediatric psychology. 3rd edition. New York: Gilford; 2003. p. 119–40.

16. Miller VA, Drotar D. Discrepancies between mother and adolescent perceptions of diabetes-related decision-making autonomy and their relationship to diabetes-related conflict and adherence to treatment. J Pediatr Psychol 2003;28: 265–74.

17. Holmbeck GN, Devine KA. Psychosocial and family functioning in spina bifida. Dev Disabil Res Rev 2010;16:40–6.

18. McDonnell GV, McCann JP. Why do adults with spina bifida and hydrocephalus die? A clinic-based study. Eur J Pediatr Surg 2000;1(Suppl 10):31–2.

19. Singhal B, Mathew KM. Factors affecting mortality and morbidity in adult spina bifida. Eur J Pediatr Surg 1999;1(Suppl 9):31–2.

20. McGuire EJ, Woodside JR, Borden TA, et al. Prognostic value of urodynamic testing in myelodysplastic patients. J Urol 1981;126:205–9.

21. McGuire EJ, Woodside JR. Diagnostic advantages of fluoroscopic monitoring during urodynamic evaluation. J Urol 1981;125:830–4.

22. Bauer SB. Management of neurogenic bladder dysfunction in children. J Urol 1984;132:544–5.

23. Bauer SB, Hallett M, Khoshbin S, et al. Predictive value of urodynamic evaluation in newborns with myelodysplasia. JAMA 1984;252:650–2.

24. Mickelson J, Cheng E, Yerkes E. Urologic issues of the pediatric spina bifida patient: a review of the genitourinary concerns and urologic care during childhood and adolescence. J Pediatr Rehabil Med 2009;2:51–9 An interdisciplinary Approach.

25. Clayton DB, Brock JW 3rd. Urologist's role in the management of spina bifid: a continuum of care. Urology 2010;76:32–8. DOI: 10.1016/j.urology.2009.12.063. Available at: http://sciencedirect.comlibproxy.usc.edu/science?_ob=articleURL&B6VJW. Accessed May 31, 2010.

26. Joseph DB, Bauer SB, Colodny AH, et al. Clean intermittent catheterization in infants with neurogenic bladder. Pediatrics 1989;4984:78–82.

27. Schlager TA, Clark M, Anderson S. Effects of a single use sterile catheter for each void on the frequency of bacteriuria in children with neurogenic bladder on intermittent catheterization for bladder emptying. Pediatrics 2001;108:E71.
28. Lapides J, Diokno AC, Silber SJ, et al. Clean, intermittent self-catheterization in the treatment of urinary tract disease. J Urol 1972;107:458–61.
29. Koff SA. Guidelines to determine the size and shape of intestinal segments used for reconstruction. J Urol 1988;140:1150–1.
30. Koff SA. The shape of intestinal segments used for reconstruction. J Urol (Paris) 1988;94:201–3.
31. Walker RD 3rd, Flack CE, Hawkins-Lee B, et al. Rectus fascial wrap: early results of a modification of the rectus fascial sling. J Urol 1995;154:771–4.
32. Mitrofanoff P. Trans-appendicular continent cystostomy in the management of the neurogenic bladder. Chir Pediatr 1980;21:297–305.
33. Shapiro SR, Johnston JH. The results of conservative management of neurogenic vesical dysfunction in children. Prog Pediatr Surg 1977;10:185–95.
34. Gonzalez R, Schimke C. Strategies in urologic reconstruction in myelomeningo-coele. Curr Opin Urol 2002;12:485–90.
35. Metcalfe PD, Cain MP, Kaefer M, et al. What is the need for additional bladder surgery after bladder augmentation in childhood? J Urol 2006;176:1801–5 [discussion: 1805].
36. Nguyen HT, Baskin LS. The outcome of bladder neck closure in children with severe urinary incontinence. J Urol 2003;169:1114–6.
37. Landau EH, Gofrit ON, Pode D, et al. Bladder neck closure in children: a decade of followup. J Urol 2009;182:1797–801.
38. Gerharz EW, Eiser C, Woodhouse CR. Current approaches to assessing the quality of life in children and adolescents. Br J Urol 2003;97:150–4.
39. Parkin PC, Kirpalani HM, Rosenbaum PL, et al. Development of a health-related quality of life instrument for use in children with spina bifida. Qual Life Res 1997;6: 123–32.
40. Eiser E, Morse R. A review of measures of quality of life for children with chronic illness. Arch Dis Child 2001;84:205–11.
41. McCormick MC, Charney EB, Stemler MM. Assessing the impact of a child with spina bifida on the family. Dev Med Child Neurol 1986;28:53–61.
42. Mobley CE, Harless LS, Miller KL. Self-perceptions of preschool children with spina bifida. J Pediatr Nurs 1996;11:217–24.
43. Brown J. Toilet training the child with spina bifida. Fact Sheet Series. Washington, DC: Spina Bifida Association; 2005.
44. World Health Organization. In: Promoting the development of infants and young children with spina bifida and hydrocephalus: a guide for mid-level rehabilitation workers, 62. Geneva: World Health Organization; 1996. Available at: http://whqlibdoc.who.int/hq/1996/WHO_RHB_96.5.pdf. Accessed May 29, 2010.
45. Merkens M, Spina Bifida Association's Professional Advisory Council. Guidelines for spina bifida health care services throughout the lifespan. 3rd edition. Washington: Spina Bifida Association; 2006.
46. Moore C, Kogan BA, Parekh A. Impact of urinary incontinence on self-concept in children with spina bifida. J Urol 2004;171:1659–62.
47. Impact of child sexual abuse. National resource center on child sexual abuse 1992. Available at: http://www.prevent-abuse-now.com/stats.htm. Accessed May 30, 2010.

48. Rajmil L, Herdman M, Fernandez de Sanmamed M, et al. The Kidscreen Group Generic health-related quality of life instruments in children and adolescents: a qualitative analysis of content. J Adolesc Health 2004;34:37–45.

49. Sawin KJ, Brei TJ, Buran CF, et al. Factors associated with quality of life in adolescents with spina bifida. J Holist Nurs 2002;20:279–304.

50. Sawin KJ, Buran CF, Brei TJ, et al. Correlates of functional status, self-management, and developmental competence outcomes in adolescents with spina bifida. SCI Nurs 2003;20(2):72–85.

51. Sawin KJ, Bellin MH, Roux G, et al. The experience of parenting an adolescent with spina bifida. Rehabil Nurs 2003;28(6):173–85.

52. Buran CF, Sawin KJ, Brei TJ, et al. Adolescents with myelomeningocele: activities, beliefs, expectations, and perceptions. Dev Med Child Neurol 2004;46:244–52.

53. Buran CF, McDaniel AM, Brei TJ. Needs assessment in a spina bifida program: a comparison of the perceptions by adolescents with spina bifida and their parents. Clin Nurse Spec 2002;16:256–62.

54. Stepansky MA, Roache CR, Holmbeck GN, et al. Medical adherence in young adolescents with spina bifida: longitudinal associations with family functioning. J Pediatr Psychol 2010;35:167–76.

55. Wysocki T, Taylor A, Hough BS, et al. Deviation from developmentally appropriate self-care autonomy: association with diabetes outcomes. Diabetes Care 1996;19: 119–25.

56. Holmbeck GN, Johnson SZ, Wills K, et al. Observed and perceived parental overprotection in relation to psychosocial adjustment in pre-adolescents with a physical disability: the mediational role of behavioral autonomy. J Consult Clin Psychol 2002;70:96–110.

57. Dicianno BF, Kurowski BG, Young JM, et al. Rehabilitation and medical management of the adult with spina bifida. Am J Phys Med Rehabil 2008;87(12):1027–50.

58. Cahill RA, Kiely EA. The spectrum of urological disease in patients with spina bifida. Ir J Med Sci 2003;172:180–4.

59. Verhoef M, Lurvink M, Barf HA, et al. High prevalence of incontinence among young adults with spina bifida: description, prediction and problem perception. Spinal Cord 2005;43:331–40.

60. Lemelle JL, Guillemin F, Aubert D, et al. Quality of life and continence in patients with spina bifida. Qual Life Res 2006;14:1481–92.

61. Neville-Jan A. The problem with prevention: the case of spina bifida. Am J Occup Ther 2005;59:527–39.

62. Iezzoni L. When walking fails: mobility problems of adults with chronic conditions. Berkeley (CA): University of California Press; 2003.

63. Cardenas DD, Topolski TD, White CJ, et al. Sexual functioning in adolescents and young adults with spina bifida. Arch Phys Med Rehabil 2008;89:31–5.

64. Gatti C, Del Rossi C, Ferrari A, et al. Predictors of successful sexual partnering of adults with spina bifida. J Urol 2009;182:1911–6.

65. Culleres GR, Sugranes JC, Fina AC, et al. Sexuality and urinary incontinence among 143 patients with spina bifida: a randomly prospective study. Arch Phys Med Rehabil 2008;89:E133 (Poster 342).

66. Buffart LM, Nan Den Berg-Emons R, Van Meeteren JV, et al. Lifestyle, participation, and health-related quality of life in adolescents and young adults with myelomeningocele. Dev Med Child Neurol 2009;51:886–94.

67. Hunt GM, Oakeshott P. Outcome in people with open spina bifida at age 35: prospective community based cohort study. BMJ 2003;326:1365–6.

68. Fletcher JM, Brei TJ. Introduction: spina bifida - a multidisciplinary perspective. Dev Disabil Res Rev 2010;16:1–5.
69. Plunkett JM, Braren V. Five-year experience with clean intermittent catheterization in children. Urology 1982;XX(2):128–30.
70. Tarnowski KJ, Drabman RS. Teaching intermittent self-catheterization skills to mentally retarded children. Res Dev Disabil 1987;8:521–9.
71. Katrancha ED. Clean intermittent catheterization in the school setting. J Sch Nurs 2008;24(4):197–204. Available at: http://jsn.sagepub.com. Accessed May 31, 2010.
72. Tait AR, Voepel-Lewis T, Malviya S. Do they understand? (Part II): assent of children participating in clinical anesthesia and surgery research. Anesthesiology 2003;98:609–14.

Achieving Continence with a Neurogenic Bowel

Susan R. Leibold, RN, MSN, CNS-P, CDDN

KEYWORDS

• Neurogenic bowel • Spina bifida • Continence
• Suppository • Enema

This article reviews the developmental considerations involved in helping the family of a child with spina bifida who needs to achieve bowel continence. Strategies for success based on an algorithm are interwoven throughout the discussion. The current medications and techniques used at the developmentally appropriate times designed for optimal success are presented.

OVERVIEW

A hallmark in every young family's life is toilet training and eliminating diapers. Parents of a newborn with spina bifida have no idea what to expect or how to parent an infant with a disability. Lack of knowledge can lead to anxiety and a crisis of confidence in the parent.

Toilet training is a watershed event in a young family's life. Bowel continence is a critically important aspect of adaptive function with enormous implications for the future. Bowel accidents are embarrassing and lead to social isolation, affecting peer relations and social success. They affect the work environment and may be a barrier to employment. Incontinence may have a lasting impact on friendships and intimacy.

Research has identified several issues related to incontinence in adults, including the decreased participation due to the time programs take, a sense of helplessness when the program did not work, the shame when asking others for assistance, and the social isolation if accidents occurred.[1] Adults with spina bifida have felt the loss of the pediatric clinic, with no identified resource for assistance in the adult health care community.

Quality-of-life (QOL) studies have attempted to evaluate the impact of achieving continence in a person's life.[2,3] Adults and teenagers with spina bifida have a lower health-related QOL score than matched controls. The effect of urinary versus fecal continence on QOL was difficult to separate. Surgical intervention, although effective

Developmental Disabilities, Texas Scottish Rite Hospital for Children, 2222 Welborn Street, Dallas, TX 75219, USA
E-mail address: Sue.leibold@tsrh.org

Pediatr Clin N Am 57 (2010) 1013–1025
doi:10.1016/j.pcl.2010.08.002
0031-3955/10/$ – see front matter © 2010 Elsevier Inc. All rights reserved.

in achieving continence, did not affect the health-related QOL. The developmental age when bowel continence was acquired has not been evaluated in relation to its impact on the QOL of the teenager/adult with spina bifida. Regardless, continence is clearly one important aspect of health-related QOL in those with spina bifida.

PATHOPHYSIOLOGY OF THE NEUROGENIC BOWEL

Bowel movements occur through the combined activity of colonic motility, rectal storage, and elimination. The neurologic innervations of the colon include the sympathetic nervous system from T10 through L2 (inhibitory impulses in the colon and rectum), the parasympathetic system from S2 through S4 (stimulatory innervation to the descending colon and rectum), and the enteric nervous system contained in the intestinal wall regulating colorectal motility.[4,5]

Liquid feces enter the ascending colon and move through the colon by contractions and mixing of the contents. This promotes absorption of water to form solid stool as it passes through the descending colon. The rectum's main function is to store feces, and it requires the ability to be relaxed until a certain amount of stool has filled the rectal vault. The internal sphincter remains closed through inhibitory impulses and has brief moments of relaxation, releasing gas. The internal sphincter relaxes (parasympathetic response) as the rectal vault reaches a certain volume and stool begins to move through it. The external sphincter's parasympathetic stimulation controls the stools' passage or containment. The neurogenic bowel has one or more of these components interrupted.[6]

In children with spina bifida, most lesions are above the S2 level, resulting in a neurogenic bowel. Colonic motility is not related to level of lesion or mobility and is prolonged as compared with controls.[7] Slow colonic transit is related to symptoms of constipation and fecal impaction. The inability to sense impending bowel movements or to "hold it" results in fecal incontinence.

DEVELOPMENTAL ASPECTS OF BOWEL CONTROL

Infants have several stools throughout a 24-hour period. Stools are seedy, loose, and soft until solid food is introduced. The frequency decreases to 1 to 2 stools per day as babies approach their first birthday. At about 18 months of age, the stool becomes more formed. At 2 years, the child becomes more aware of having had a stool. Toilet training ensues as the toddler becomes aware of impending stools and chooses to use the toilet or not. By age 4 years, most children are toilet trained and cleaning themselves.[8]

Infants with spina bifida tend to experience constipation as solid foods are introduced. Prevention of constipation is helpful in later development of a continence program.[9] Lack of rectal awareness and lack of sensation in the perineal/buttock area results in stool remaining in the diaper until odor brings attention to its presence. Cleaning and changing remain in the parental domain as the child enters school. Continence programs need to begin at the developmentally appropriate age, to assist children with spina bifida in reaching similar developmental milestones to their unaffected peers.

TYPES OF BOWEL CONTINENCE PROGRAMS
Dietary

Fluid and fiber remains the foundation for prevention of constipation and treatment of continence. The intake amount is determined by age and weight.[10] In infants, fluid and baby fruits are key. In older children, fiber is added through cereals, fruits, vegetables, and breads/grains. Parents are taught to read labels to identify higher-fiber foods. Whole-grain products, introduced before low-fiber refined products, can be well-accepted by children as they grow. Fluid goals are determined by weight in children younger than 10 years. For those older than 10 years, 64 ounces a day is the basic goal. Fiber goals are based on the age plus 5 to 10 (3 years + 5 = 8 g of fiber a day).[11] Children with spina bifida have a Chiari II malformation and may exhibit dysphagia demonstrated by low fluid volumes and difficulty with food textures. Evaluation and intervention with dietary and oral motor therapy may be helpful.

Dietary triggers that cause an unexpected or loose stool need to be identified as the child is introduced to new foods. Chocolate and spicy and greasy foods can cause loose stools. Foods that contain corn or high-fructose corn syrup are especially implicated in causing loose or unexpected stools. Some children are more sensitive than others. Any child that has not had formed stools needs to have a diet history taken to identify possible food triggers.

Medications

Oral medications are used to promote a soft formed stool that is in the rectal vault at the time planned by the family/teenager for a bowel movement. Osmotic and bulk laxatives are effective in keeping the stool soft and formed when diet and liquids are not enough. A stimulant laxative, such as senna, strengthens colonic motility, enabling the stool to be in the rectal vault 6 hours (typically) after ingestion and providing predictability for elimination. When used with a suppository or enema program, individuals can be continent (**Table 1**).

Suppositories

Suppository programs are designed to produce a bowel movement within a few minutes of insertion. Liquid glycerin, liquid glycerin with docusate (mini-enema), and bisacodyl in a wax or water-soluble base are currently available (**Table 2**). The liquid suppositories require holding the external sphincter shut after the liquid is inserted for a few minutes to stimulate emptying. In the author's clinical experience, this is easier for a parent to do with a baby or toddler but difficult for an older child to do independently while sitting on the toilet.

The bisacodyl suppository needs to be inserted through the internal anal sphincter and not into stool. The wax-based suppository is difficult to time and may work in 15 or 45 minutes. The water-based suppository works in about 5 minutes and is easy for a school-aged child or teenager to insert on the toilet and have a bowel movement in 5 to 10 minutes.

Difficulties arise with either suppository if there is low rectal tone. The anal canal has loose tissue, making it challenging to insert the suppository (liquid or solid) through the loose tissue to the internal anal sphincter and rectal vault. A clue to the problem is a parent reporting that no suppository works, an indicator for use of the cone enema.

Enema Programs

Cone enemas (transanal) use a colostomy irrigation system, which administers 1 to 2 cups of tap water while sitting on the toilet. The cone acts as a plug to keep the water inside. It produces significant rectal distention and, once removed, results in a bowel movement being completed in 20 minutes. These enemas are very effective and can be used independently by teenagers with sacral level 1 to lumbar level 1 spina bifida (sitting balance is important).[12,13]

Table 1
Oral maintenance medications

Common Use	Medications	Actions	Dose	Comments
Maintenance Oral	Lactulose	Poorly absorbed sugar with osmotic effect	Infant: 2.5–10 mL/d Child: 7.5 mL/d	Gas and bloating can be common side effects
	Senna (8.6 mg/5 ml = 1 tab) Pedia-Lax senna (1 strip = 8.6 mg senna)	Stimulant laxative Grape-flavored quick-dissolving strips	Infant: 1.25–2.5 mL/d 1–5 y: 2.5–10 mL/d >6 y: 5–15 mL/d	Produces peristalsis; works usually in 6 h from ingestion
	Psyllium- (Perdiem, Fiberall)	Bulk laxative	Titrate	May cause bloating; must take with plenty of water to avoid intestinal obstruction
	Polycarbophil (Fibercon, Equalactin, Konsyl)	Bulk laxative	Titrate	Synthetic fiber resistant to bacterial degradation = less bloating; helpful in regulating fluid excess in bowel
	Guar gum (Benefiber)	Bulk laxative	1 scoop = 3 g fiber; increase as needed every 3 days	Taste-free, grit-free; does not thicken or alter taste or texture of food
	Polyethylene glycol 3350 (MiraLax)	Osmotic laxative	0.8 g/kg once/d	Not as effective in neurogenic bowel; difficult to time; can cause gas bloating and nausea
	Metoclopramide (Reglan)	Motility agent-gastro/colonic	0.1–0.2 mg/kg 2–3 times/d	Decreases time stool sits in colon and prevents constipation
	Erythromycin	Motility agent-gastro/colonic	2–3 mg/kg/dose 3 times/d	Decreases time stool sits in colon

Common Use	Medications	Actions	Dose	Comments
Maintenance Rectal	Docusate (Enemeez [4 mL of docusate, glycerin, polyethylene glycol])	Stimulant	Contents of 1 mini enema; If added to transanal or MACE irrigation solution may add 1–2	Difficult to hold in with incompetent external sphincter—does not support independence Assist in speed of emptying; administration technique supports independence
	Bisacodyl-rectal suppository (Magic Bullet [bisacodyl in water base])	Stimulant	1 suppository inserted on toilet	Can be done independently; works in 5–10 min

Table 2
Maintenance medications

Abbreviation: MACE, Malone antegrade continence enema.

The antegrade continence enema (ACE) or Malone antegrade continence enema (MACE) is a surgical intervention that creates a continent channel at the ascending colon near the cecum. Tap water with or without other stimulants is run through, flushing out the entire colon. The MACE can be used independently by older school-aged children and teenagers.[14] The time can be problematic, taking an average of 53 minutes. There can be "wash out" failure allowing for the water to move around the stool and not push the stool with it. Long-term follow-up indicates a 40% dropout rate in adulthood, which may be related to the lack of support in maintaining a bowel management program in the transition to adult care. Stomal stenosis may occur, requiring surgical revision.[15] Despite many of these concerns, there remains a high degree of contentment.

A variation on this is the placement of a tube such as the Chait Trapdoor (Cook, Bloomington, IN, USA),[16] which is similar to a gastrostomy (g-) tube (has a balloon on the tube end that is inserted into the stomach) but has a coil on the end inserted into the ascending colon to anchor it. The Chait Trapdoor is opened to insert a catheter and run the solution through the colon. The Chait Trapdoor can be done through interventional radiology as opposed to a surgery needed to create the continent stoma.

The left antegrade continent enema[17] is a continent channel created in the left abdomen into the descending colon and acts like antegrade cone, eliminating the stool in the descending colon. The average transit time is 31 minutes and requires less solution to be instilled. The occurrence of stomal stenosis is 50% less than with the ACE.

Colostomies are not currently used unless there is a malformation of the rectum. They can be effective for some families, providing a measure of control and eventual independence.

There are no published reports on the use of the sacral nerve stimulator in the spina bifida or pediatric population, but it may have some future possibilities. The sacral nerve stimulator has electrodes implanted into the S2-4 anterior nerve roots, which are controlled by an external transmitter to stimulate the anal-rectal area so that evacuation occurs. The sacral nerve stimulator has been used and evaluated in adults with spinal cord injury. The results in this population indicate an improvement in constipation, increased defecation frequency, reduced defecation time, reduction in the number of medications required previously, and high degree of patient satisfaction.[18]

GOALS OF A BOWEL CONTINENCE PROGRAM

The goals of a bowel program need to be developmentally based and adjusted for independence as the child grows. This may necessitate interventions with adaptive toileting equipment or enlargement of the bathroom and entrance for a wheelchair. Flexibility is also important. Family routines differ from the working week to the weekend, and by adjusting the time that oral medications are given, the time of elimination is adjusted.

Bowel programs taking only 20 to 30 minutes can be fit into a daily routine and have a greater compliance as children enter their teenage years (**Table 3**).

PLANNING A BOWEL PROGRAM

Assessment is the cornerstone of determining a bowel program because each child is different, and for a program to be successful, it needs to be individualized. At Texas Scottish Rite Hospital for Children, a 13-point assessment has been developed that assists with planning a bowel program for achieving continence. The program still requires initial adjustment of medications or timing and troubleshooting with changes of routine. Parents can be reassured that their first actions are not in vain, and minor adjustments continue to help them move toward their goal (**Table 4**).[19]

Assessment frequently identifies constipation. "Clean-out" is needed before starting a continence program. The use of oral and rectal medications can prevent cramping and discomfort. The rectal vault has the hardest stool, and use of an enema is the first step. Oral medications move the stool around to the rectal vault. If there are balls of stool throughout, starting with mineral oil for lubrication is helpful. The clean-out is successful when the stool is liquid (**Table 5**).

DEVELOPMENTAL CONSIDERATIONS IN BOWEL CONTINENCE PROGRAMS

In 1998, Texas Scottish Rite Hospital developed an algorithm to assist with planning a bowel continence program that provides a family with the greatest success in achieving continence (**Fig. 1**).

Infancy

The transactional model of development[20] is a useful construct for pediatricians to use when considering how to support parents and their infants with spina bifida. Briefly, this approach suggests that the infant, the caregiver, and the environmental context surrounding them are all active players in the child's developmental and behavioral

Table 3
Goals of a bowel continence program

Goal	Factors
Time	20–30 minutes is easily incorporated into a daily routine
Flexibility	It can be done at camp, on vacation, in college, or adjusted from school days to weekends
Independence	Program is adjusted as the child grows, transferring the program from the parent to the school-aged child/teenager

Table 4
Assessment of neurogenic bowel

Assessment	Rationale	Treatment Options
Stool Form	Balls indicate slow motility and too much water being absorbed. Oatmeal consistency indicates increased motility and the need for bulking.	Clean out old hard stool; assess fiber and fluid intake and adjust them. Assess foods that may increase motility.
Stool Consistency	Hard or formed or soft	Fluid and/or fiber goals / Fiber supplements, motility aids
Stool Amount	4-6 in for 3-6-year-olds / 6-8 in for 6-8-year-olds / 8-10 in for 9-11-year-olds / 12-18 in for 12 years and older	Emptying typical amount for age ensures descending colon is empty and prevents constipation
Tone of Anal Canal	If there is good tone to the internal anal sphincter, it responds to a suppository.	If it does not respond to a suppository or fleet enema, check rectal tone.
Level of Paraplegia	Ease of transfer to toilet; ability to balance on toilet	Ability to balance works with a suppository or enema; ability to transfer, ability to follow an enema program (cone or ACE)
Age	<5 years / >6 years	Parent-dependent / Work toward independent program
Mobility	Wheelchair fits into bathroom	If not, work on a program using a bedside commode
Fluid	Provides the liquid to keep stool soft.	If cannot meet fluid goals, may indicate dysphagia
Fiber	Adequate intake bulks stool and form is easier to eliminate	Introduce supplements if cannot eat target goals
Medications	Anticholinergics slow smooth muscle and contribute to constipation. Anesthetics slow motility.	Plan to counteract when beginning anticholinergics or anticipating surgery
Family Routines	Can schedule activities and have flexibility to adjust	Assist parents with more support when they require exact plans to follow.
Programs Attempted in the Past	Families may be resistant to trying again when *nothing has worked.*	Families need to know that a bowel management program is inclusive and includes fluid, fiber, medications, and timing of elimination.
Learning Issues	Executive function can pose problems to adjusting bowel program for changes in routine or weather.	Work with early teenagers to start assessing their output and what adjustments need to occur in situations that they encounter.

Table 5
Medications for bowel clean-out

Common Use	Medications	Action	Dose	Comments
Clean-out Oral	Polyethylene glycol	Osmotic laxative	2–11 y: 8.5 g (halfway to measuring line in 4 oz liquid) >12 y: 17 g in 8 oz of liquid	Disimpaction
	Mineral oil	Lubricant	5–11 y: 5–15 mL 1–3 times/d >12 y: 30–60 mL 1–3 times/d	Do not use if suspect aspiration; long-term use loses fat-soluble vitamins; may break down g-tube
	Milk of magnesia	Osmotic laxative	<2 y: 0.5 mL/kg/dose 2–5 y: 5–15 mL/d, once or in divided doses 6–11 y: 15–30 mL/d or in divided doses >12 y: 30–60 mL/d, once or in divided doses	Also in chewable form
	Magnesium citrate	Osmotic laxative	<6 yr: 2–4 mL/kg, once or divided 6–12 y: 100–150 mL >12 y: 150–300 mL	Do not use in patients with renal insufficiency
Clean-out Rectal	Phospho-soda enema	Osmotic effect in intestine by drawing water into lumen of the gut, producing distension, promoting peristalsis, and evacuation	2–11 y: contents of one 2.25-oz pediatric enema >12 y: contents of one 4.5-oz adult enema	Not for use in patients with renal insufficiency Do not exceed more than 1/d
	Fleet mineral oil enema	Ease elimination of stool, decreasing water absorption and lubricating rectum	2–11 y: 30–60 mL as single dose >12 y: 60–150 mL as single dose	Used with significant hard stool in rectal vault; difficult to keep in with incompetent sphincter Safe for children with renal insufficiency
	Milk and molasses enema	Osmotic effect without a shift in electrolytes	<8 y: equal parts milk and molasses (1oz:1oz; 2oz:2oz) 8 y–teenaged: 4–8 oz milk and 4–8 oz molasses	Safe for patients with renal insufficiency

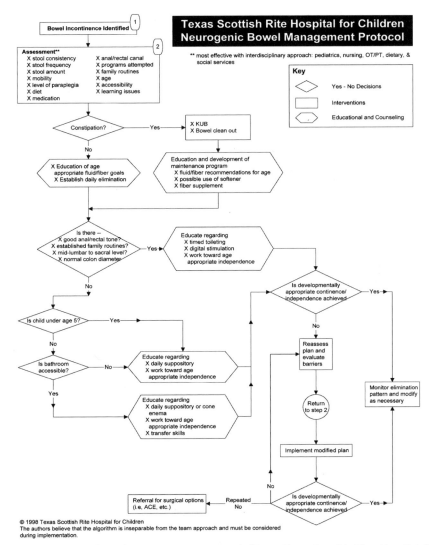

Fig. 1. Neurogenic bowel management protocol. (*From* Texas Scottish Rite Hospital for Children; with permission.)

growth. The interaction is a dynamic, organic process that alters each of the afore-mentioned players.

This is especially true in a situation as complex as the delivery, neonatal surgery, rehabilitation, and ultimate normalization of activities that occur in these infants and their families. Attachment issues on the part of the infant and the caregiver are potential risk factors, especially as they affect feeding and elimination in the infant with Chiari II malformations. Underlying neurodevelopmental differences in the infant can create real or perceived feeding issues and a sense of concern regarding self-competency in the parents.

What would otherwise seem to be the *simple acts of feeding and defecating* can create questions of health, well-being, competency, and emotional well-being for the infant-parent dyad. Even the ability to adequately handle a diaper rash can be a challenge, because the acidic stool *burns* the skin in an insensate area without infants *communicating* their needs to the parent.

Thus, what would otherwise be considered typical infant care can create barriers to the natural attachment of infant to parent, because caution, worry, and competence remain daily issues. The child-health profession (eg, physician, nurse) must have awareness and understanding of these dynamics to avoid contributing to the tension experienced in families of infants with spina bifida. Supporting the family with suggestions of adding juice or lactulose enhance parent competence if stools become pasty (like peanut butter) or ball-shaped and difficult to push out, whereas polyethylene glycol can cause diarrhea and adding fiber may cause increased gas and bloating, resulting in infant discomfort and parent stress. Understanding and patience in this pivotal developmental period can reap rewards for years to come for the family and the professionals supporting them.

Toddler/Preschooler

The goal at this age is to learn independence, and toilet training is one of the tasks needed to achieve this goal. Children with spina bifida lack the sensation to know when they have had a bowel movement in their diaper. Creating the opportunity for choosing to sit on the potty-chair provides experience in asserting independence. Toilet training may be facilitated by the following:

- Clean out hard stool if necessary, and maintain soft stools with fluids, fiber, and polyelthylene glycol or lactulose if necessary.
- Identify when/if the toddler has a daily bowel movement.
- If no regular emptying time exists, begin giving senna syrup, a natural vegetable laxative that can be timed to predict when a bowel movement would occur. It works in 6 hours. Using a liquid suppository at the 6-hour mark triggers an emptying, assisting with toilet training because the child has predictable stool. Fluid and fiber need to be included in the daily routine. Lactulose can be added if fiber intake is low.
- All changing of diapers should be in the bathroom by this age to teach that all bladder/bowel emptying occurs there. The potty-chair should be available and offered to the toddler after the suppository is administered. Making the choice of where to have the bowel movement becomes the child's.
- As children grow, including them in making choices with foods and fluids begins to lay the ground work for decision-making in the future.

School Age

The challenges for school-aged children are to expand their world outside the family home. Making friends and exploring interests in the community are important for future independent life. Participation may be threatened if a child has bowel accidents. Parental anxiety can undermine the child's emerging sense of autonomy and competence. Guidance needs to be provided to transition the bowel program to one that can eventually be followed by the older child.

- If the child is using a liquid suppository, change to a solid suppository, which can be inserted on the toilet.
- Accessibility to the toilet affects the degree of independence with a continence program. Bathroom doorways can be a huge barrier if a child is a full-time

wheelchair user, which may necessitate the parent carrying the child into the bathroom. Transfers from wheelchair to toilet are the next step for independence.
- If there is low rectal tone or continued bowel accidents on the suppository program, the cone enema can be very effective.

Surgical intervention with creation of a stoma in the right ascending or left descending colon is the next step if the cone enema is not effective. Accessibility to the bathroom and onto the toilet is important in this program as well. Most children are able to learn to do this independently.

Adolescence

Independence and identity are the important goals in the teenager. Teenagers may begin to question why they must do all the health routines asked of them in a day. Nonadherence to a continence program may be an expression of adolescent rebellion. Helping teenagers to develop a basic understanding of their spina bifida provides a basis for the self-care regimen suggested by the health care team. Developing social activities with other teenagers with spina bifida creates a normalizing environment in which continence programs are perceived as normal and acceptable. Bowel programs may go awry because teenagers decrease fluid intake to reduce the frequency of catheterization, refuse high-fiber foods, choose not to follow the bowel program, or forget to take their medicines, and so forth. A supportive and structured environment helps to reduce many of these behaviors.

Table 6
Troubleshooting

Problem	Suggestions
Stools without time to sit	Lower dose of oral medication. Response to oral medication may be quicker and the time needs to be moved closer to the elimination time. Evaluate diet for high-fructose corn syrup or other food triggers.
Stools after finishing	Consider adding fiber supplement to bulk up stool. Increase physical activity before timed evacuation. Change mechanism of eliminating (from suppository to transanal enema)
Stools begin hard and become loose	Evaluate water intake and increase if needed. Evaluate mechanism for emptying and change program if needed. Evaluate for high-fructose corn syrup.
Stools when walking	Use of transanal enema assists in emptying the descending colon and preventing ambulation stools.
Teenage girls with liquid stool once a month	Assess if associated with monthly period; if so, give quarter dose of medications used for diarrhea. If not associated with cycles, evaluate for impaction or constipation.
Cannot meet fluid goals	Evaluate for dysphagia related to the Chiari II malformation.
Cone enema leaks while water is instilling	Anal canal dilates reflexively with fluid; wiggle cone in for a tighter seal.

- Use of a weekly medication box showing multiple times of the day is helpful in remembering and checking on the medication use. This can be filled weekly together with the parent and eventually become the responsibility of the teenager.
- Place all of the bathroom equipment conveniently close to the toilet. Parents have placed gloves, lubricant, suppositories/enema, and personal wipes and disinfectant wipes for equipment in plastic drawers next to the toilet. A small covered disposal unit can mask odors from others using the bathroom.[21,22]
- Use fiber supplements so that teenagers eat similar food to their peers. Encouraging fluid intake at catheterization and mealtimes helps teenagers develop healthy habits that can be carried into adulthood.
- Design bowel programs for the teenager to do independently. Working with an occupational therapist may be helpful to identify adaptations and equipment.

TROUBLESHOOTING

After deciding on the initial program, all bowel programs require adjustment. More fiber may be needed for improved stool consistency. A range of possible senna or polyethylene glycol doses allows parents to adjust the dose based on daily diet and fluid intake. Surgery causes constipation from the anesthesia and/or pain medication. Adjustments before and after surgery minimize constipation. Helping parents identify progress is important when adjustments are needed (**Table 6**).

SUMMARY

Achieving an effective bowel continence program requires support for the family in areas of bowel management, medication adjustment, dietary triggers, fluid/fiber goals, and adaptive equipment use. The Spina Bifida Association has an excellent manual on bowel management,[12] with helpful guides for many of the continence techniques. Helping families understand that continence is an achievable goal is very important when facing the future and the transition of children into adulthood. The understanding and support provided by the primary care doctor to the family is invaluable in achieving lifelong success.

REFERENCES

1. Johnsen V, Skattebu E, Aamot-Andersen A, et al. Problematic aspects of faecal incontinence according to the experience of adults with spina bifida. J Rehabil Med 2009;41:506–11.
2. Lemelle JL, Guillemin F, Aubert D, et al. Quality of life and continence in patients with spina bifida. Qual Life Res 2006;15:1481–92.
3. Nanigian DK, Nguyen T, Tanaka ST, et al. Development and validation of the fecal incontinence and constipation quality of life measure in children with spina bifida. J Urol 2008;180:1770–3.
4. Krogh K, Christensen P. Neurogenic colorectal and pelvic floor dysfunction. Best Pract Res Clin Gastroenterol 2005;23:531–43.
5. Cheetham MJ, Malouf AJ, Kamm MA. Fecal incontinence. Gastroenterol Clin North Am 2001;30(1):115–30.
6. Krogh K, Christensen P, Laurberg S. Colorectal symptoms in patients with neurological diseases. Acta Neurol Scand 2001;103:335–43.
7. Pigeon N, Leroi AM, Devroede G, et al. Colonic transit time in patients with myelomeningocele. Neurogastroenterol Motil 1997;9:63–70.

8. Dunn AM. Elimination pattern. In: Burns CE, Barber N, Brady MA, et al, editors. Pediatric primary care: a handbook for nurse practitioners. Philadelphia: W.B. Saunders Company; 1996. p. 277–87.

9. Leibold S. A systematic approach to bowel continence for children with spina bifida. Eur J Pediatr Surg 1991;1(1):23–4.

10. Feinberg AN, Feinberg LA, Atay OK. Gastrointestinal care of children and adolescents with developmental disabilities. In: Greydanus DE, Patel DR, Pratt HD, editors. Pediatr Clin N Am. Philadelphia: W.B. Saunders Company; 2008;55(6):1343–58.

11. Chad H-C, Lai M-W, Chen S-Y, et al. Cutoff volume of dietary fiber to ameliorate constipation in children. J Pediatr 2008;153(1):45–9.

12. Braun PG, Brown JP, Leibold S, et al. Bowel management and spina bifida [booklet]. Washington, DC: Spina Bifida Assoc; 2009. p. 1–50.

13. Ausili E, Focarelli B, Tabacco F, et al. Transanal irrigation in myelomeningocele children: an alternative, safe and valid approach for neurogenic constipation. Spinal Cord 2010;48:560–5.

14. Jinbo AK. The challenge of obtaining continence in a child with a neurogenic bowel disorder. J Wound Ostomy Continence Nurs 2004;31:336–50.

15. Yardley IE, Pauniaho S-L, Baillie CT, et al. After the honeymoon comes divorce: long-term use of the antegrade continence enema procedure. J Pediatr Surg 2009;44:1274–7.

16. Yamout SZ, Glick PL, Lee Y-H, et al. Initial experience with laparoscopic Chait Trapdoor™ cecostomy catheter placement for the management of fecal incontinence in children: outcomes and lessons learned. Pediatr Surg Int 2009;25:1081–5.

17. Sinha CK, Butler C, Haddad M. Left antegrade continent enema (LACE): review of the literature. Eur J Pediatr Surg 2008;18:215–8.

18. Valles M, Rodriguez A, Borau A, et al. Effect of sacral anterior root stimulator on bowel dysfunction in patients with spinal cord injury. Dis Colon Rectum 2009;52(5):986–92.

19. Leibold S, Ekmark E, Adams R. Decision-making for a successful bowel continence program. Eur J Pediatr Surg 2000;10(1):26–30.

20. Sameroff AJ, Chandler MJ. Perinatal risk and the continuum of caretaking causalty. In: Horowitz F, Hetherington M, Scarr-Salaptaek S, editors. Review of child development research, vol 4. Chicago: University of Chicago Press; 1975. p. 187–244.

21. Velde SV, Van Biervliet S, Van Renterghem K, et al. Achieving fecal continence in patients with spina bifida: a descriptive cohort study. J Urol 2007;178:2640–4.

22. Leibold S. Neurogenic bowel and continence programs for the individual with spina bifida. J Pediatr Rehabil Med 2008;1:325–36.

Cultural Considerations in the Care of Children with Spina Bifida

Kathryn Smith, RN, MN[a,b,c],*, Kurt A. Freeman, PhD[d],
Ann Neville-Jan, PhD, OTR/L[e], Stacey Mizokawa, PhD[f],
Elizabeth Adams, PhD, RD[g]

KEYWORDS

- Spina bifida • Culture • Latin American • Hispanic
- Folic acid • Neural tube defects

Spina bifida occurs when the neural tube fails to close during early fetal development. This failure results in a vast array of potential impairments.[1] Malformations such as these are called neural tube defects (NTDs), which are structural abnormalities of the brain and vertebral column.[2] According to the Centers for Disease Control and Prevention (CDC) National Center on Birth Defects and Developmental Disabilities,[3] each year in the United States approximately 3000 infants are born with spina bifida or other NTDs. The Spina Bifida Association[4] estimates that 70,000 people in the United States are currently living with spina bifida; however, spina bifida is considered underreported on birth certificates according to birth certificate data from the National Vital Statistics System, a part of the CDC National Center for Health Statistics, so this estimate is believed to be considerably low.[5]

[a] Department of Pediatrics, University Center for Excellence in Developmental Disabilities, University of Southern California, 4650 Sunset Boulevard, MS #53, Los Angeles, CA 90027, USA
[b] Division of General Pediatrics, Spina Bifida Center, Childrens Hospital Los Angeles, 4650 Sunset Boulevard, MS #53, Los Angeles, CA 90027, USA
[c] Department of Pediatrics, Keck School of Medicine USC, 4650 Sunset Boulevard, MS #53, Los Angeles, CA 90027, USA
[d] Division of Psychology, Child Development & Rehabilitation Center, Oregon Health & Science University, PO Box 574, Portland, OR 97207-0574, USA
[e] Department of Occupational Science & Occupational Therapy, University of Southern California, 1540 Alcazar Street, CHP-133, Los Angeles, CA 90089, USA
[f] Division of General Pediatrics, University Center for Excellence in Developmental Disabilities, Childrens Hospital Los Angeles, University of Southern California, 4650 Sunset Boulevard, MS #53, Los Angeles, CA 90027, USA
[g] Department of Public Health and Preventive Medicine, Oregon Health & Science University, 707 SW Gaines Road, Portland, OR 97239, USA
* Corresponding author. Department of Pediatrics, Keck School of Medicine USC, 4650 Sunset Boulevard, MS #53, Los Angeles, CA 90027.
E-mail address: kasmith@chla.usc.edu

Pediatr Clin N Am 57 (2010) 1027–1040
doi:10.1016/j.pcl.2010.07.019   pediatric.theclinics.com
0031-3955/10/$ – see front matter © 2010 Published by Elsevier Inc.

Although the causes of spina bifida are not fully understood, scientists believe that both genetic and environmental factors act simultaneously to cause this and other NTDs. However, 95% of babies with spina bifida and other NTDs are born to parents with no family history of such conditions.[2] The CDC reports that spina bifida and other NTDs occur more frequently in some ethnic groups than others. For example, NTDs are more common in Hispanics than in individuals of other ethnicities.[3]

Individuals with spina bifida live with a range of disabilities depending on the level of their lesion. Common conditions that affect those with spina bifida are sensory and motor impairment, bowel and bladder incontinence, hydrocephalus, learning and developmental delays, and orthopedic problems.[6] Persons with spina bifida often undergo numerous surgeries, and experience multiple providers and interventions. Research has shown that individuals living with spina bifida can thrive with the help of a multidisciplinary team of specialists that can manage and tend to their individual needs.[6]

Ethnic minorities make up a large portion of the population of individuals with spina bifida, and cultural beliefs may affect the use of health care and influence behavior in relation to modifying risk factors for spina bifida. In considering culture, ethnicity, and spina bifida, this article (1) reviews the literature that addresses the prevalence of spina bifida related to different ethnic groups, (2) identifies factors that intersect with prevalence, and (3) discusses implications for clinical practice. Because "… culture and language may affect health, healing and wellness belief systems; how illness, disease, and their causes are perceived; the behaviors of individuals seeking health care; and the delivery of health care services and provider behavior",[7] consideration of culture becomes a critical component of the care of individuals with spina bifida and their families.

The Institute of Medicine's (IOM)[8] report on health disparities, Unequal Treatment, defines culture as "the accumulated store of shared values, ideas (attitudes, beliefs, values, and norms), understandings, symbols, material products and practices of a group of people"[(p523)]. Ethnicity refers to a "shared culture and way of life, especially as reflected in language, folkways, religious and other institutional forms, material culture such as clothing and food, and cultural products such as music, literature, and art"[(p523)]. Race connotes "a concept wherein groups of people sharing certain physical characteristics are treated differently based on stereotypical thinking, discriminatory institutions and social structures, a shared worldview, and social myths"[(p525)]. There is no scientific evidence for a category such as race based on physical characteristics or genetics. The American Anthropological Association (AAA), in comments to the Interagency Committee to the Census Bureau, recommends that race and ethnicity be combined into a category race/ethnicity. For future consideration, they recommend that race be eliminated from government documents. Further, the AAA delineates ethnicity or ethnic group as social categories more important for scientific purposes.[9]

The United States is increasingly multicultural and diverse. As a result, it is becoming more difficult to categorize individuals into a single racial/ethnic group. Federal census categories have changed over the years, and other federal agencies, such as the CDC and National Institutes for Health, as well as business and industry, change their practices to use updated categories. Since 2000, residents of the United States have been allowed to indicate more than 1 race/ethnicity on the census. As a result, health care research often uses the concepts of culture, ethnicity, and race in confounding and opposing ways, which adds confusion when investigating trends across various studies as well as over time. In an attempt to provide some clarity and consistency, this article primarily uses the term ethnicity as defined by the IOM and avoids using race unless part of a particular study.

THE INTERSECTIONS OF RACE, ETHNICITY, AND CULTURE ON SPINA BIFIDA
Prevalence Data

The prevalence of spina bifida for the latest available reporting period (2003–2005) using data from national samples of birth certificates is 1.90 per 10,000 live births; 2.0 per 10,000 live births among infants with non-Hispanic white mothers, 1.96 among infants with Hispanic mothers, and 1.74 among infants with non-Hispanic black mothers.[10] In this report, the prevalence of spina bifida was similar for infants born to Hispanic and non-Hispanic white mothers, contrary to findings identified by others that demonstrated a higher prevalence among Hispanic women than women in other racial/ethnic groups both before and after folic acid fortification. Previous research found notable differences in prevalence rates of NTDs, including spina bifida, across different ethnic/racial groups. Specifically, prevalence has been shown to be approximately 50% to 100% higher among Hispanic women compared with non-Hispanic white women,[11–16] and women of African American and Asian descent seem to have the lowest prevalence of spina bifida. The overrepresentation of NTDs generally, and spina bifida specifically, among Hispanic populations in the United States has been stable.

Prevention and Folic Acid

Given differential prevalence rates, research on cultural, ethnic, and racial issues in spina bifida and NTDs has focused almost exclusively on individuals of Hispanic descent. This article reviews current literature on changing patterns of birth rates, and demographic, cultural, and acculturation factors that affect the expression of spina bifida.

Since the mid to late 1990s, a dramatic and notable decrease in the rate of NTDs has been observed in the United States. This change has been accounted for almost exclusively by changes in access to dietary and supplemental folic acid. In 1992, the US Public Health Service recommended that all women of childbearing age consume 400 μg of folic acid daily to help prevent NTDs, estimating that 50% to 70% of NTDs could be prevented through daily consumption of this amount of folic acid.[17] In 1996, the US Food and Drug Administration mandated the addition of folic acid to all enriched cereal grain products by January of 1998.[18] The timing and implementation of mandated fortification created opportunities to investigate the prevalence of spina bifida and other NTDs before and after mandated fortification.

Multiple studies show that fortification dramatically reduced the prevalence of NTDs.[15,19–23] Although folic acid fortification clearly results in decreased NTDs, reductions in births following mandatory fortification do not seem comparable across ethnic groups. Williams and colleagues[15] examined the decline in the prevalence of spina bifida during the transition to mandatory folic acid fortification in the United States from 1995 to 2002. They found that the prevalence of spina bifida per 10,000 live births was highest among Hispanic births at all 3 time points (January 1995–December 1996, 6.49; January 1997–September 1998, 5.52; October 1998–December 2002, 4.18), followed by non-Hispanic white births (1995–1996, 5.13; 1998–1998, 4.37; 1998–2002, 3.37), with the lowest prevalence among non-Hispanic black births (1995–1996, 3.57; 1997–1998, 2.53; 1998–2002, 2.90). Folic acid fortification was also associated with a significant decrease in the prevalence of spina bifida in non-Hispanic white and Hispanic births. However, the magnitude of reduction in NTD births was markedly lower among African Americans, and the change was not statistically significant. Reasons for these differences across African American and other groups are not fully understood; the lower basal rate of NTDs in African Americans may account for this finding.

Although existing research shows that folic acid supplementation reduces rates of NTDs among Hispanic people comparable with reductions observed in non-Hispanic white people, rates remain notably higher among Hispanic people even after fortification. Given this, attempts have been made to elucidate the factors that account for discrepancies across ethnic groups. Some research suggests that differences in folic acid consumption patterns account for continued high rates of NTDs among Hispanic people. Hispanic women may be less likely to use folic acid supplements,[24] and Spanish-speaking women may be less likely to take preconception multivitamins[25] compared with English-speaking women. Hispanic women living along the Mexican-American border have been shown to have low rates of folic acid supplementation, with the primary source from vitamins[26]; supplementation via vitamins may not be as effective as dietary folic acid because less of the folate is bioavailable.[27] Hispanic women have also been shown to be less likely to consume breakfast cereals,[28] which are high in fortified folic acid.

Several lines of evidence suggest that differences in folic acid consumption do not account for differences in NTD rates. African American women have been shown to consume even less folic acid through supplements and dietary intake than Hispanic women.[29,30] Similar serum folate levels have been found among Hispanic and African American women before and after fortification became mandatory.[17]

Harris and Shaw[31] suggested that factors such as ethnic/racial differences in sensitivity to folate, genetic factors, or other unknown factors may account for observed differences. Ethnic differences exist in methylenetetrahydrofolate reductase gene polymorphisms,[32] which regulate folate distributions. Specifically, 1 of 2 polymorphisms of the methylenetetrahydrofolate reductase gene (C677T), which may be associated with increased risk of NTDs, was highest in Hispanic women and lowest in African American women.

Maternal weight status has also been shown to affect risk for having a child with an NTD. Specifically, women who are obese seem to have almost twice the risk,[33–35] even after controlling for race.[33] This is relevant because some research suggests that Hispanic women may have higher visceral adipose tissue and total fat percentage for body mass index than African American and white women.[36,37] Thus, although prevalence of prepregnancy obesity has been shown to be higher in African American women compared with white and Hispanic women,[38] the type and percentage of fat tissue is greater for Hispanic women, which may help explain the increased prevalence of NTDs among children of Hispanic descent. Poor weight gain[39] or weight loss early in pregnancy[40] has been associated with increased risk of NTDs, although this seems to be independent of race/ethnicity.[39]

Acculturation and other demographic variables that may affect rates of NTDs among Hispanic mothers have been more thoroughly studied. Several investigations have been conducted to determine whether foreign-born versus United States–born Hispanic women experience different rates of NTDs. Using data gathered from 1997 to 2003 via the National Birth Defects Prevention Study, Ramadhani and colleagues[41] showed that Hispanic mothers born in Mexico/Central America were 50% more likely to have births of spina bifida than their United States–born counterparts. They also noted that there were no differences in rates of folic acid use between United States–born and foreign-born mothers, providing further evidence that folic acid may not be the most critical variable explaining higher rates of NTDs among Hispanic women. Canfield and colleagues[42] also found an association between birth status of mothers and risk of NTD in offspring. Specifically, they noted that the greatest risk for birth of a child affected by spina bifida occurred among foreign-born Hispanic women in the United States for less than 5 years. They found no increased risk for having a birth with spina bifida or anencephaly for United States–born Hispanic women compared with white women. Similar findings were noted by Velie and colleagues,[43] who showed a twofold increased risk for spina bifida among women born in Mexico but in the United States for less than 2 years, as well as relative risk among second- and third-generation women of Mexican heritage similar to that of non-Hispanic white women.

Research on the association between acculturation variables and risk of having a child with an NTD has not been consistent. For instance, Ramadhani and colleagues[41] found that foreign-born Hispanic women who had been in the United States for longer than 5 years had a higher risk of spina bifida birth than their counter- parts who were foreign-born but had been in the United States for less than 5 years. Carmichael and colleagues[16] showed that Hispanic women born in the United States who preferred to speak Spanish, used as a marker of acculturation, had lower risk of spina bifida birth than foreign-born Hispanic women regardless of language prefer- ence, United States–born Hispanic women who preferred English, and white women.

Socioeconomic variables also seem to be associated with relative risk of having a child with an NTD. Mothers with the highest income, regardless of ethnic status, may be markedly less likely to have a child with spina bifida.[42] Canfield and colleagues showed that highly educated Hispanic and white women had a 76% and 35% lower risk of have spina bifida offspring, respectively. Demographic, socioeconomic, and educational status also seem to intersect with folic acid supplementation in a way that is relevant for understanding discrepancies in births affected by spina bifida across ethnic groups. Specifically, younger women, those with less formal education, and those with lower annual household income are also less likely to take folic acid supplements daily.[44] This is important given evidence that recent immigrants to the United States are more likely to be young, less educated, and have lower incomes.[46] Research shows that folic acid supplementation rates have decreased over time for women who are Hispanic and of lower education.[46]

Cultural Factors That May Affect Care

In addition to differential prevalence rates and factors associated with biomedical and demographic risks for spina bifida, a variety of other cultural influences affect the care of children and adults with spina bifida and their families. These influences include reli- gion, the nature of relationships with providers, language differences, health literacy, and expectations regarding goals for independence.

Religion

Religion often plays a significant role in people's lives, especially as they cope with their own or family members' chronic condition. Johnstone and colleagues[47] identified that both religion and spirituality are important coping strategies for those with disabil- ities, and, in a study of quality of life for families of children with disabilities, Poston and Turnbull[48] found that families identified the importance of spirituality in their lives. In a study by Treloar,[49] individuals with disabilities and their family members described how they used their spiritual beliefs to establish meaning for disability and to respond to associated challenges, and found that participants' spiritual beliefs stabilized their lives, provided meaning for the experience of disability, and assisted with coping. In research into the association of religious and spiritual coping with well-being in Latin American people caring for older relatives with disabilities, Herrera and colleagues[50] found that intrinsic and organizational religiosity was associated with lower perceived burden, whereas nonorganizational religiosity was associated with poorer mental health. Given the importance of religion, notably among the Hispanic/Latin American, and African American communities, careful attention to an individual's or family's connection with religious and/or spiritual beliefs and practices is important for understanding factors that may assist or hinder coping.

Relationships with providers

Latin American patients tend to view clinicians as important authority figures, expecting both an expert and a friend they can talk to, and the impersonal characteristics that may accompany the typical clinical encounter are not acceptable in the Latin American culture.[51] Disparities in health outcomes among minority and racial groups are well documented[8] and are at times attributable to breakdown in the quality of the clinician-patient relationship. Cooper and colleagues[52] described several elements of the clinician-patient relationship that may be affected by race/ethnicity, including communication, partnership, respect, knowing, affiliation/liking, and trust. Race, ethnicity, and language substantially influence the quality of the doctor-patient relationship, and minority patients, especially non–English speakers, are less likely to engender an empathic response from providers and be encouraged to participate in decision making.[53] Others have found that race-concordant visits (in which patient and provider are the same race) result in higher ratings of patient satisfaction than race-discordant visits, were longer, had a more positive patient affect, and improved continuity of care.[52] The clinician-patient relationship is strengthened when patients see themselves as similar to their clinicians and this is associated with higher ratings of trust, satisfaction, and intention to adhere.[54] These findings have significant implications for spina bifida programs in which large groups of minority patients may be seen, with care provided by nonminority, English-speaking providers. Because long-term adherence to medical procedures is required to promote health and minimize complications associated with spina bifida, the nature of the clinician-patient relationship may have a significant effect on outcomes and quality of life. To our knowledge, specific study of the clinician-patient relationship in spina bifida has not been conducted, and this area warrants future research.

Language differences

Although it may be helpful if health care providers share a common cultural and linguistic background with their patients, this is not always possible and, some argue, does not necessarily mean that culturally appropriate care is being provided.[55] However, when the patient and health care provider speak different languages, the use of interpreters to facilitate communication is among the most basic of recommendations typically made.[51,56,57] Research has shown that having interpreters facilitate communication with health care providers can increase willingness to seek health care, improve satisfaction with the services provided, increase treatment adherence, and improve health outcomes for non–English speakers.[56] Although more costly, medical interpreters should be offered to the patient and family, rather than ad hoc interpreters (such as other hospital staff or family members).[51,58] Although both trained medical interpreters and ad hoc interpreters make similar types of interpreting errors, the errors made by ad hoc interpreters can be significantly more likely to have possible clinical consequences than the errors made by trained interpreters.[59] In addition, the use of children or adolescents as interpreters must be avoided, because it places such a heavy emotional burden on them and could also disrupt the parent-child relationship.

Even when the language barrier can be bridged with the assistance of an interpreter, cultural variations can still interfere with communication between a patient and the medical providers. Singleton and Krause[60] provided several examples of how cultural expectations may interfere with effective communication, including a cultural tendency to avoid conflict causing patients to agree to participate in treatments that they do not agree with or understand; a cultural preference for obtaining information from a male provider, meaning that important information provided by a female clinician may be dismissed; and self-advocacy being frowned on in some cultures, so patients may not ask questions even when an interpreter is available.

Health literacy
In addition to the language spoken by the patient and the family, the level of literacy in English and the primary language must also be considered.[60] Health education materials are often provided in a written format and may use sophisticated language that may be difficult to understand, or the materials may have been written in a manner that reflects American traditions and beliefs, without accounting for cultural differences, thus making the content less accessible for some cultural groups even when translated into different languages.

Health literacy must also be considered in the care of individuals with spina bifida and their families. Healthy People 2010[61] defines health literacy as "the degree to which individuals have the capacity to obtain, process, and understand basic health information and services needed to make appropriate health decisions." As such, health literacy includes the ability to understand instructions on prescription drug bottles, appointment slips, health education materials, instructions, and consent forms, and the ability to negotiate complex health care systems. Being health literate requires a complex group of reading, listening, analytical, and decision-making skills, and the ability to apply these skills to health situations. According to the American Medical Association,[62] poor health literacy is "a stronger predictor of a person's health than age, income, employment status, education level, and race" and the IOM[8] reports that 90 million people in the United States (nearly half the population) have difficulty understanding and using health information. Patients and family members are often provided with written instructions related to care for individuals with spina bifida. If not well written and geared toward the health literacy level of the target population, the material is not helpful, and may provide a false sense of security among caregivers that transmitted information is being understood.

Goals for independence
We have observed that cultural influences affect a family's feelings about promoting independence in the child or youth with spina bifida, at times causing tension with providers seeking to support independence and self-care. Typical areas of dissension include self-catheterization, bowel management, independence in the community, planning for independent living and careers, and social and romantic relationships.[63]

The issue of independence has not been well addressed in the literature, particularly as it relates to cultural differences. We were able to locate only 1 study in a search of MEDLINE and PsychINFO from 1995 to the present that addressed ethnicity and spina bifida (one of several health conditions studied) other than in relation to prevalence or prevention. Wolman and colleagues[64] conducted a qualitative study of the wishes and expectations of 63 parents from diverse cultural backgrounds for their children (5–12 years of age) with chronic illnesses. The most common primary diagnoses of the 63 children included asthma,[9] cerebral palsy,[8] seizure disorder,[8] diabetes mellitus,[7] and spina bifida.[6] Participants self-identified as African American,[20] Hispanic,[19] and

European American.[21] Using a content analysis approach, researchers learned that, regardless of ethnicity, the parents' most frequently expressed wish was that their children's condition be cured or improved. Next, parents wished for their children to be healthy and happy. Wishes related to independent living, financial independence, and the ability to drive a car were exclusively expressed by parents of children with mental retardation and mobility impairments. "Studying well, having a good education, and staying in school" and behavioral concerns such as "I hope she will stop being demanding"[(p269)] and "that he could get along with his brother harmoniously, just minor disagreements"[(p270)] were the wishes mentioned primarily by African American and Hispanic parents, regardless of condition. Many parents were not able to state expectations and were worried or fearful about the future.

Some specific cross-cultural/ethnic differences were observed in the Wolman and colleagues[64] study. For instance, African American and Hispanic parents' expectations differed notably from European American parents in concerns about social issues such as violence and risky behaviors. However, the investigators suggested that cultural/ethnic differences may not be the primary reason for such differences. Specifically, they note that, rather than being a unique effect of ethnicity, this difference could be interpreted as a combination of minority status, low income, and socioeconomic status. There was a significant difference in income between African American and Hispanic participants compared with European American participants. They suggested that wishes and expectations related to independent living were related to condition rather than ethnicity. However, more research needs to be conducted to understand whether differences in cultural practices (eg, tendency of children to remain in parental home until marriage) also relate to issues such as independent living more than socioeconomic or other related variables.

IMPLICATIONS FOR CLINICAL PRACTICE

Culture matters when health professionals conduct assessments and recommend treatment of patients who have spina bifida in hospitals and outpatient clinics. Culture matters not in an essentialist way such that ethnicity, race, or language defines a particular culture. For example, when clinicians make statements or operate with beliefs that ascribe attributes or behavioral patterns based on overt markers of presumed cultural affiliation (eg, making generalized assumptions that "African Americans believe...thus, my African American patient must also believe..."), they are attending to a superficial, and perhaps stereotypical, perspective on culture. Culture matters in a more complex manner in terms of how a person lives their life and what is personally important regarding illness or disability.

The concept of culture originated within the discipline of anthropology, and the study has evolved over time from the singular investigation of the culture of small villages to studies of the culture of various socially constructed groups of individuals, including urban neighborhoods, hospitals, and clinics. This broadening of the concept of culture is not so much about a place as an encounter. Mattingly[65] refers to the clinic as a border zone where professional and patient cultures meet and negotiate, and, as such, has the potential for either negatively or positively affecting what happens during the encounter and after. In the discussion of the role of culture in the interaction between clinician and patient, Mattingly stated that "In this hybrid place...cultural identities are reinvented in unexpected ways and belonging is marked by liminality and contestation rather than any uncomplicated citizenship"[(p139)]. In this view of culture, clinical encounters are areas of friction, tension, and conflict. Lawlor[66] presented an alternative view that clinician-patient encounters are "moments of meeting…jointly constructed, complementary actions in which each participant contributes something unique and there is a shared state of consciousness"[(p308)].

Most of the research literature about spina bifida refers to ethnicity and race, and pays little attention to culture, with perhaps the exception being the small body of literature investigating the association between acculturation and risk of NTDs. Kleinman and Benson[67] stated that, although there are "culturally informed therapeutic strategies" used in clinic settings, there is a lack of evidence to support such practices. Thus, despite increased attention to cultural competence within medical and allied health professions, as well as calls for culturally informed practices, virtually no empirical evidence exists to guide clinicians.

As an alternative to cultural competence, Kleinman and Benson[68] propose a reformulation of culture for clinicians that would replace the traditional traits-list approach to cultural competence that frequently occurs in clinical thinking. This new formulation uses an explanatory models approach, first introduced by Kleinman[67] in an earlier work, as a way to improve medical education. Kleinman[67] defines explanatory models as "…the notions that patients, families, and practitioners have about a specific illness episode"[(p121)]. This approach, taught in many medical schools across the United States, uses an informal interview or what Kleinman[67] calls a miniethnography as a way of understanding the illness experience from the perspective of the patient and family.

Kleinman and Benson[68] outline a series of 6 steps for clinicians to consider in this revised approach to cultural competence:

1. Understand how the individual patient's ethnic identity may be relevant to the clinical situation. What does the patient and family view as the problem? What is their explanatory model?
2. Determine what is at stake for the patient and family as they confront the illness. What are the consequences of the illness for them?
3. Construct the illness narrative. This comprises a sequence of questions to more thoroughly ascertain the patient and family explanatory model (eg, What do they call this problem? What does it do to their body? What are their fears about the illness and the treatment?).
4. Identify stresses and supports that may be connected to the illness and interventions. What tensions are related to work, financial issues, and so forth?
5. Reflect on how the patient's culture might influence the clinical relationship. What are the clinicians' biases about the specific illness?
6. Question the approach taken to intervention. Does this treatment work in this specific case?

These steps serve only as guides, and Kleinman and Benson[67] emphasize that explanatory models are amorphous. They change with time and with the chaos that surrounds the illness experience. Therefore they need to be frequently revisited and revised.

Given the evidence supporting a reduction in the prevalence of spina bifida through use of folic acid before and early in pregnancy, every effort should be made to provide this information to women, especially those of Hispanic heritage. Hispanic women are less likely than other women to take multivitamins,[69] an important source of fortification, hence targeted education efforts must be developed to address concerns about vitamin use, as well as providing information about folate-rich foods. Educational programs are likely to be most effective if they are linked to cultural eating practices, and fortified foods that may fit within traditional food preferences must be identified. Given that foreign-born Hispanic women[41,43] and those with less education and from lower socioeconomic status[43] are at greater risk for having children with NTDs, educational efforts should be developed to specifically target these groups. This strategy is particularly important given that educational attainment and socioeconomic status are positively corrected with rates of folic acid supplementation.[45] In addition, evidence points to maternal obesity and diabetes as a risk factors for NTDs[33-35]; coordinated efforts that address obesity, diabetes control or prevention, and preconception folate fortification and consumption of a folate-rich diet are likely to be the most appropriate means of addressing multiple risk factors for NTDs.

Given the importance of outreach and education to reduce the risk of NTDs, there is a need to continue to work with primary care and women's health providers to address educational needs and develop strategies and interventions intended to reach high-risk populations. Strategies such as the use of prometoras (ie, an outreach worker in a Hispanic community who is responsible for raising awareness of health and educational issues), working with faith-based organizations, and other outreach efforts designed to meet women in the communities in which they live can help achieve educational goals. Although community-based efforts may be highly appropriate for dissemination of information and education, it is important to be mindful of the potential challenges of doing so. For example, it is possible that women may not be interested in receiving information about reproduction within church or other public/community settings.

As identified earlier, several cultural factors can influence care for the patient with spina bifida and his or her family, including religion, relationships with providers, language differences, literacy and health literacy, and expectations regarding independence. Providers can build on the support offered by religion or spirituality by inquiring about beliefs, recognizing their importance to the patient and family, and providing opportunity for discussion about needs and concerns. Many facilities have pastoral staff or counselors who can assist individuals during stressful times, or when questions arise about spiritual issues related to disability. Further investigation into the effect of religion and spirituality on the care of individuals with spina bifida would aid in providing appropriate support in this area.

Enhancing relationships between providers, patients, and families is important to ensuring the long-term success of the treatment plan, achievement of patient goals, and positive health outcomes. Clinician skilled in patient-centered care who show respect and support patient involvement can overcome issues of race to forge a strong connection with patients, leading to greater patient satisfaction, trust, and commitment to treatment.[54] A more diverse clinician workforce has been suggested as a way to enhance the clinician-patient relationship. Provider training in cultural competence and self-awareness has been suggested, but there are limited studies suggesting the usefulness of this approach, and the suggestion for training patients to be more assertive has also been made.[53]

Language differences can be addressed through the use of well-trained interpreters; multilingual spoken, visual, and written educational materials; and bilingual staff. Educational materials should be provided at a variety of educational levels, and tested on target audiences to obtain feedback and validate the item's usefulness.

The goal of independence and successful transition to adulthood for children and youths with spina bifida should be addressed early, and age-appropriate participation in care should be promoted. Young children can be encouraged to participate in self-care procedures by such simple activities as opening the catheter package for the parent. Similarly, parents can describe care while they are providing it, such as the reasons for, and findings of, skin checks, to share information with the child, model appropriate care, and set the stage for transition to health self-management when possible. The Life Course Model described in other articles in this issue includes culture as a significant environmental factor in the life course of a child with spina bifida. At every stage of development, this influence is important in determining how the child and family are able to stay on a trajectory to the desired outcome of full participation in important functional domains, including health self-management, personal relationships, and employment. Providers and families can use the Life Course Model to monitor progress and make changes as needed to increase the chances of desirable outcomes. Providers can explore with families the meaning of the disability within the cultural context, as well as long-term goals for the child and beliefs about independence. Conflicts in beliefs can then be brought to the team and shared to seek resolution and optimal health and well-being for the patient.

Research related to culture, race, and ethnicity has focused on prevalence and prevention. Although these are important areas of study, we argue that the aim of researchers and policymakers in this area should include both prevention, improvement in the quality of life, and the goal of full participation for children and adults with spina bifida.

ACKNOWLEDGMENTS

The authors gratefully acknowledge the work of Marianne Ward and Kristy Macias in the preparation of this manuscript.

REFERENCES

1. Cabrera RM, Hill DS, Etheredge AJ, et al. Investigations into the etiology of neural tube defects. Birth Defects Res C Embryo Today 2004;72(4):330–44.
2. American College of Obstetricians and Gynecologists. Neural tube defects. Obstet Gynecol 2003;102(1):203–13 ACOG Practice Bulletin No 44. Available at: http://www.greenjournal.org/cgi/reprint/102/1/203.pdf. Accessed March 28, 2008.
3. Center for Disease Control and Prevention-National Center on Birth Defects and Developmental Disabilities. Folic acid: frequently asked questions. Available at: http://www.cdc.gov/ncbddd/folicacid/faqs.htm#baby; 2008. Accessed March 27, 2008.
4. Spina Bifida Association. How many people in the United States are there with spina bifida. Available at: http://www.spinabifidaassociation.org/site/c. liKWL7PLLrF/b.2700311/k.13CB/How_Many_People_With_Spina_Bifida_In_The_US.htm; 2008. Accessed March 28, 2008.
5. Mathews TJ. National Center for Health Statistics: trends in spina bifida and anencephalus in the United States 1991–2005. Available at: http://www.cdc.gov/nchs/products/pubs/pubd/hestats/spine_anen.htm; 2007. Accessed April 1, 2008.
6. Sander A. Living with spina bifida: a guide for families and professionals (preface). Chapel Hill (NC): The University of North Carolina Press; 2004.
7. Office of disease prevention and health promotion. Available at: http://odphp.osophs.dhhs.gov/projects/healthcomm/objective2.htm. Accessed May 5, 2010.
8. Smedley B, Stith A, Nelson A. Unequal treatment: confronting racial and ethnic disparities in health care. Washington, DC: Institute of Medicine/National Academies Press; 2003.
9. American Anthropological Association. A brief history of the OMB Directive. Available at: http://www.aaanet.org/gvt/ombdraft.htm; 1997. Accessed April 5, 2010.

10. Boulet SL, Gambrell D, Shin M, et al. Racial/ethnic differences in the birth prevalence of spina bifida - United States. MMWR Morb Mortal Wkly Rep 2009;57: 1409–13.
11. Feuchtbaum LB, Currier RJ, Riggle S, et al. Neural tube defect prevalence in California (1990–1994): eliciting patterns by type of defect and maternal race/ethnicity. Genet Test 1999;3:265–72.
12. Shaw GM, Jensvold NG, Wasserman CR, et al. Epidemiologic characteristics of phenotypically distinct neural tube defects among 0.7 million California births, 1983–1987. Teratology 1994;49:143–9.
13. Canfield MA, Annegers JF, Brender JD, et al. Hispanic origin and neural tube defects in Houston/Harris County, Texas. I. Descriptive epidemiology. Am J Epidemiol 1996;143:1–11.
14. Canfield MA, Honein MA, Yuskiv N, et al. National estimates and race/ethnic-specific variation of selected birth defects in the United States, 1999–2001. Birth Defects Res A Clin Mol Teratol 2006;76:747–56.
15. Williams LJ, Rasmussen SA, Flores A, et al. Decline in the prevalence of spina bifida and anencephaly by race/ethnicity: 1995–2002. Pediatrics 2005;116:580–6.
16. Carmichael SL, Shaw GM, Song J, et al. Markers of acculturation and risk of NTDs among Hispanic women in California. Birth Defects Res A Clin Mol Teratol 2008;82:755–62.
17. Centers for Disease Control and Prevention. Folate status in women of childbearing age, by race/ethnicity–United States, 1999–2000. MMWR Morb Mortal Wkly Rep 2002;51:808–10.
18. Boulet SL, Yang Q, Mai C, et al. Trends in the postfortification prevalence of spina bifida and anencephaly in the United States. Birth Defects Res A Clin Mol Teratol 2008;82(7):527–32.
19. Centers for Disease Control and Prevention. Spina bifida and anencephaly before and after folic acid mandate—United States, 1995–1996 and 1999–2000. MMWR Morb Mortal Wkly Rep 2004;53:362–5.
20. Honein MA, Paulozzi LJ, Mathews TJ, et al. Impact of folic acid fortification of the US food supply on the occurrence of neural tube defects. JAMA 2001;285: 2981–6.
21. Mathews TJ, Honein MA, Erickson JD. Spina bifida and anencephaly prevalence—United States, 1991–2001. MMWR Morb Mortal Wkly Rep 2002;51:9–11.
22. Williams LJ, Mai CT, Edmonds LD, et al. Prevalence of spina bifida and anencephaly during the transition to mandatory folic acid fortification in the United States. Teratology 2002;66:33–9.
23. Centers for Disease Control and Prevention. QuickStats, spina bifida and anencephaly rates - United States, 1991, 1995, 2000, and 2005. MMWR Morb Mortal Wkly Rep 2008;57:15. Available at: http://www.cdc.gov/mmwr/PDF/wk/mm5701. pdf. Accessed April 1, 2010.
24. Ahluwalia IB, Lyon DK. Are women with recent live births aware of the benefits of folic acid? MMWR Morb Mortal Wkly Rep 2001;50:3–14.
25. Perlow JH. Comparative use and knowledge of preconceptional folic acid among Spanish- and English-speaking patient populations in Phoenix and Yuma, Arizona. Am J Obstet Gynecol 2001;184:1263–6.
26. Suarez L, Hendricks KA, Cooper SP, et al. Neural tube defects among Mexican Americans living on the US-Mexico border: effects of folic acid and dietary folate. Am J Epidemiol 2000;152:1017–23.
27. Rose NC, Mennuti MT. Periconceptional folic acid supplementation as a social intervention. Semin Perinatol 1995;19:243–54.

28. Siega-Riz AM, Popkin BM, Carson T. Differences in food patterns at breakfast by sociodemographic characteristics among a nationally representative sample of adults in the United States. Prev Med 2000;30:415–24.
29. Jasti S, Siega-Riz AM, Bentley ME. Dietary supplement use in the context of health disparities: cultural, ethnic and demographic determinants of use. J Nutr 2003;133:2010S–3S.
30. Ford ES, Ballew C. Dietary folate intake in US adults: findings from the third National Health and Nutrition Examination Survey. Ethn Dis 1998;8:299–305.
31. Harris JA, Shaw GM. Neural tube defects: why are rates high among populations of Mexican descent? Environ Health Perspect 1995;103:163–4.
32. Esfahani ST, Cogger EA, Caudill MA. Heterogeneity in the prevalence of methylenetetrahydrofolate reductase gene polymorphisms in women of different ethnic groups. J Am Diet Assoc 2003;103:200–7.
33. Waller D, Mills J, Simpson J. Are obese women at higher risk for producing malformed offspring? Am J Obstet Gynecol 1994;170:541–8.
34. Waller DK, Shaw GM, Rasmussen SA, et al. Prepregnancy obesity as a risk factor for structural birth defects. Arch Pediatr Adolesc Med 2007;161:745–50.
35. Watkins M, Scanlon K, Mulinare J, et al. Is maternal obesity a risk factor for anencephaly and spina bifida? Epidemiology 1996;7:507–12.
36. Carroll JF, Chiapa AL, Rodriquez M, et al. Visceral fat, waist circumference, and BMI: impact of race/ethnicity. Obesity (Silver Spring) 2008;16:600–7.
37. Fernández JR, Heo M, Heymsfield SB, et al. Is percentage body fat differentially related to body mass index in Hispanic Americans, African Americans, and European Americans? Am J Clin Nutr 2003;77:71–5.
38. Chu SY, Kim SY, Bish CL. Prepregnancy obesity prevalence in the United States, 2004–2005. Matern Child Health J 2009;13(5):614–20.
39. Siega-Riz AM, Hobel CJ. Predictors of poor maternal weight gain from baseline anthropometric, psychosocial, and demographic information in a Hispanic population. J Am Diet Assoc 1997;97:1264–8.
40. Robert E, Francannet C, Shaw G. Neural tube defects and maternal weight reduction in early pregnancy. Reprod Toxicol 1995;9:57–9.
41. Ramadhani T, Short V, Canfield MA, et al. Are birth defects among Hispanics related to maternal nativity or number of years lived in the United States? Birth Defects Res A Clin Mol Teratol 2009;85:755–63.
42. Canfield MA, Ramadhani TA, Shaw GM, et al. Anencephaly and spina bifida among Hispanics: maternal, sociodemographic, and acculturation factors in the National Birth Defects Prevention Study. Birth Defects Res A Clin Mol Teratol 2009;85:637–46.
43. Velie EM, Shaw GM, Malcoe LH, et al. Understanding the increased risk of neural-tube defect-affected pregnancies among Mexican-born women in California: immigration and anthropometric factors. Paediatr Perinat Epidemiol 2006;20:219–30.
44. Green-Raleigh K, Carter H, Mulinare J, et al. Trends in folic acid awareness and behavior in the United States: the Gallup organization for the march of dimes foundation surveys, 1995–2005. Matern Child Health J 2006;10(Suppl 7):177–82.
45. Dey AN, Lucas JW. Physical and mental health characteristics of U.S. and foreign-born adults: United States, 1998–2003. Adv Data 2006;369:1–19.
46. Centers for Disease Control and Prevention. Folate status in women of childbearing age, by race/ethnicity-United States, 1999–2000, 2001–2002, and 2003–2004. MMWR Morb Mortal Wkly Rep 2007;55:1377–80.

47. Johnstone B, Glass BA, Oliver RE. Religion and disability: clinical, research and training considerations for rehabilitation professionals. Disabil Rehabil 2007; 29(15):1153–63.

48. Poston DJ, Turnbull AP. Role of spirituality and religion in family quality of life for families of children with disabilities. Educ Train Dev Disabil 2004;39(2):95–108.

49. Treloar LL. Disability, spiritual beliefs and the church: the experiences of adults with disabilities and family members. J Adv Nurs 2002;40(5):594–603.

50. Herrera AP, Lee JW, Nanyonjo RD, et al. Religious coping and caregiver well-being in Mexican-American families. Aging Ment Health 2009;13(1):84–91.

51. Perez-Stable EJ. Issues in Latino health care - Medical staff conference. West J Med 1987;146:213–8.

52. Cooper LA, Roter DL, Johnson RL, et al. Patient-centered communication, ratings of care, and concordance of patient and physician race. Ann Intern Med 2003; 139:907–15.

53. Ferguson WJ, Candib LM. Culture, language, and the doctor-patient relationship. Fam Med 2002;34(5):353–61.

54. Street RL, O'Malley KJ, Cooper LA, et al. Understanding concordance in patient-physician relationships: personal and ethnic dimensions of shared identity. Ann Fam Med 2008;6(3):198–205.

55. Shaw SJ. The politics of recognition in culturally appropriate care. Med Anthropol Q 2001;19:290–309.

56. Brach C, Fraserirector I. Can cultural competency reduce racial and ethnic health disparities? A review and conceptual model. Med Care Res Rev 2000;57:181–217.

57. Shaw SJ, Huebner C, Armin J, et al. The role of culture in health literacy and chronic disease screening and management. J Immigr Minor Health 2009;11:460–7.

58. Flores G. Language barriers to health care in the United States. N Engl J Med 2006;355:229–31.

59. Flores G, Barton Laws M, Mayo SJ. Errors in medical interpretation and their potential clinical consequences in pediatric encounters. Pediatrics 2003;111:6–14.

60. Singleton K, Krause EMS. Understanding cultural and linguistic barriers to health literacy. The Online Journal of Issues in Nursing 2009;14. Manuscript 4.

61. Healthy people 2010. Available at: http://www.healthypeople.gov/. Accessed April 5, 2010.

62. AMA. Available at: http://www.ama-assn.org/. Accessed April 5, 2010.

63. Neville-Jan A, Dudgeon B, Freeman KA, et al. A qualitative study of practitioner, caregiver, and child perceptions of incontinence. Paper presented at Spina Bifida Association, First World Congress on Spina Bifida Research and Care "The Future is Now." Orlando (FL), March 15–18, 2009.

64. Wolman C, Garwick A, Kohrman C, et al. Parents' wishes and expectations for children with chronic conditions. J Dev Phys Disabil 2001;13(3):261–77.

65. Mattingly C. Reading minds and telling tales in a cultural borderland. Ethos 2008; 36(1):136–54.

66. Lawlor MC. Mothering work: negotiating health care, illness and disability, and development. In: Esdaile SA, Olson JA, editors. Mothering occupations: challenge, agency, and participation. Philadelphia: FA Davis; 2004. p. 306–23.

67. Kleinman A, Benson P. Anthropology in the clinic: the problem of cultural competency and how to fix it. PLoS Med 2006;3(10):e294.

68. Kleinman A. The illness narratives: Suffering, healing and the human condition. New York: Basic Books; 1988.

69. Thomas KB, Hauser K, Rodriguez NY, et al. Folic acid promotion for Hispanic women in Florida: a vitamin diary study. Health Educ J May 4, 2010. [Online].

Gaps and Opportunities: An Agenda for Further Research, Services, and Program Development in Spina Bifida

Kathleen J. Sawin, PhD, CPNP-PC[a],*, Cecily L. Betz, PhD, RN[b],
Ronna Linroth, PhD, OT[c]

KEYWORDS

• Spina bifida • Research • Services • Program development

GAPS AND OPPORTUNITIES IN SPINA BIFIDA RESEARCH AND PRACTICE

Both the current project to develop the Life Course Model for spina bifida, undertaken with the support of Centers for Disease Control and Prevention (CDC), and the activities of professionals in the spina bifida (SB) community[1–4] have highlighted gaps in the knowledge and programs available to individuals with SB. In 2003 CDC, the Agency for Healthcare Research and Quality (AHRQ), the National Institutes for Health, and the Department of Education sponsored a state-of-the-science consensus conference at which invited professionals presented reviews of the evidence in 16 areas and generated a research agenda (see **Table 1** for research priorities relative to the Life Course Model project.)[1] Evidenced-based guidelines for health care providers (HCPs) were developed in 2006.[4] In addition, syntheses of major focus areas in the First World Congress on Spina Bifida Research and Care further identified evidence available for practice in 2009.[2] In

[a] Children's Hospital of Wisconsin, Self-Management Science Center, College of Nursing, University of Wisconsin-Milwaukee, Box 413, Milwaukee, WI 53201, USA
[b] Department of Pediatrics, Keck School of Medicine, USC Center of Excellence in Developmental Disabilities, Children's Hospital Los Angeles, University of Southern California, 4650 Sunset Boulevard, MS# 53, Los Angeles, CA 90027, USA
[c] Adult Outpatient Services, Gillette Lifetime Specialty Healthcare Clinic, Gillette Children's Specialty Healthcare, 435 Phalen Boulevard, MN 55130, USA
* Corresponding author
E-mail address: sawin@uwm.edu

Pediatr Clin N Am 57 (2010) 1041–1057
doi:10.1016/j.pcl.2010.07.020
pediatric.theclinics.com
0031-3955/10/$ – see front matter © 2010 Elsevier Inc. All rights reserved.

Table 1
2003 research priorities[1] relative to Life Course Model Project

Domain of this Transition Project	Category from 2003 Priorities	Priorities
Self-management/health	Self-care[a]	Factors that affect the teaching and learning of self-management
		Assessment of ways to measure self-management
		Optimizing use of assistive devices
	Urology	Optional proactive therapy for urinary function
	Mobility	Optimizing mobility changes during adolescence
	Orthopedics	Prevention and management of osteoporosis
	Latex allergies	Optimal prevention management
		Latex allergy in adults
	Integument	Optimizing preventive skin care
		Optimizing treatment of skin breakdown
	Gastroenterology	Optimizing bowel management
Personal/social	Socialization	Determination of the prevalence and nature of social challenges
		Determination of risk factors (and protective factors) for impaired socialization
		Optimizing socialization
		Optimizing psychosocial development
	Sexuality	Optimizing parenting
	Family	
	Behavioral/mental health	Development of trajectories of mental health/behavioral health issues
		Optimizing mental health
Education/employment/income support	Education/employment	Factors that predict performance in school
		Participation in the labor force
		Models of transition from school to work
	Neuropsychology and learning	Evaluation of the core processing deficits
		Determination of the earliest indicators of learning difficulties
		Determination of institutional and developmental interventions that are most effective in facilitating learning
	Independence	Assessment of current functioning of adults
		Secondary conditions in adolescents and adults
		Optimizing self-determination and independence

[a] Referred to as self-management in this article.

the past 3 years, 20 professionals have also participated in the Life Course Model project described elsewhere in this issue of Pediatric Clinics of North America. The purpose of this article is to build on past work by the SB professional commu-nity[1,2,4] by discussing the gaps in the knowledge, resources, or programs available across the life course for individuals with SB identified during the development of the Life Course Model Web site.

Functioning and disability are the interaction among the health conditions and personal and environmental factors according to the International Classification of Functioning, Disability, and Health.[5] Minimizing disability-related challenges for people with SB is as important as the goal of prevention of conditions leading to SB. This analysis focuses on the 3 broad functional domains of the Life Course Model project aimed at minimizing these disability-related challenges (self-management/health, personal and social relationships, and employment/income support) and the common issues that cross these areas.

As the Life Course Model Web site was developed, strategies supported by empiric data were identified and integrated into its development. It became evident during this development process that there were gaps in the research to support the selection of empirically based clinical strategies for this resource. Most of the evidence in each of the broad functional domains is descriptive in nature, with few clinical trials establish-ing new interventions. This finding is particularly true in the personal/social relation-ships category, in which only one pilot project (n = 10) on family interventions has been reported,[6] even although this gap was identified several years ago.[7] Some prog-ress has been made in identifying learning challenges in young people with SB, espe-cially in core processing challenges and strengths.[8] However, interventions to address these challenges and build on the strengths have yet to be tested.

In this relative vacuum, important clinical programs have emerged, including a tech-nology-based transition program that has engaged young adults by focusing on building skills in transition-age young people with SB and mentoring programs,[9] the purpose of which is to enhance the development of socialization skills and those related to community integration.[10] Despite the lack of evaluation data published on these programs, they provide important options for individuals with SB when avail-able. Each of these Life Course Model domain pathways can provide relevant informa-tion for individuals with SB and their families and the HCPs who work with them. Knowledge gaps can be addressed directly with new research studies that then provide the community with evidence for practice. Simultaneously, programs can be evaluated and practice-based evidence generated that can provide useful informa-tion to the SB community and also inform future research projects. Gaps remain in both clinical programs and research; these gaps are the focus of this article.

GAPS IN RESEARCH, PROGRAMS, AND SERVICES
Health/Self-management

An abiding appreciation of and respect for the challenges families face led to the iden-tification of the need for the Life Course Model project. The research on health-related outcomes of adults with SB shows the importance of acquiring the knowledge and self-management skills necessary for health maintenance and SB condition stability. Problems in self-management can result in serious, even fatal, complications, as shown by shunt malfunctioning, impaired kidney functioning, renal failure, and pres-sure sores.[11–15] The serious and long-term consequences of these complications can be life limiting. In turn, the individual's lifestyle can be seriously affected, as shown by higher rates of unemployment and diminished ability to live independently.[13,15,16]

The evidence to inform and enlarge understanding of strategies to foster self-management/health of children with SB was reviewed and guided the development of the Life Course Model Web site to provide families with life course guidance in raising and caring for their children. Many of the recommendations provided in the self-management/health domain of the Life Course Model Web site (assessment tools, interventions, tips, resources, and referrals) were based on recommendations of clinical experts, promising practices, and theoretic rationale.

The literature on the health and self-management of children and adolescents with SB examines the phenomena from several perspectives, with noticeable gaps. The literature is characterized in part by the use of more global areas of inquiry such as adherence and independence in contrast to examining more discrete questions pertaining to central self-management tasks such as continuous intermittent catheterization (CIC). Levels of independence and adherence have been used as proxies for examining the child's self-management competencies. The studies of adherence and independence do not directly provide the evidence needed to help providers and families find the most effective instructional strategies and long-term approaches to use nor do they identify factors that facilitate or impede the acquisition of knowledge and skills needed to competently engage in SB self-management. However, these studies do provide some direction and insights to guide assessment and intervention, as presented later.

Preschool-aged and school-aged children

Having a child with SB immediately thrusts families into a new world order whose challenges seem overwhelming. These new challenges require families not only to cope with the psychosocial and economic ramifications associated with raising a child with a significant disabling condition but also to learn the surveillance and medical management skills necessary to ensure their child's physical and psychological well-being. As parents become clinically competent in managing their child's care, the process of transmitting their knowledge and skills of SB and transfer of management responsibilities to their child begins as well. For long-term management of SB, families, and eventually the child, must acquire central and peripheral sets of knowledge and skills. The central set includes the pathophysiology of SB, shunt care, CIC, bowel management, skin care, medications, and the use and maintenance of assistive devices. The peripheral set of knowledge and skills includes access to supports and resources needed for care and obtaining the health-related accommodations needed for school, work, and community living. Although empiric studies have reported findings on the medically and surgically related care for individuals with SB across the life span, there is a lack of evidence on effective instructional programs and services for parents whose children are in this age group.

During early childhood, parents are instructed by the members of the interdisciplinary team on raising and caring for their infant with SB. The professional context within which instruction takes place can positively or negatively affect parental attitudes on raising a child with SB. Parents are likely to feel overwhelmed with the new and unexpected care requirements for their child. Empathetic support coupled with patient responses to the parents' need for information about SB and its management increases parents' comfort levels, so that they ask the questions they need answered to fill in the gaps in their knowledge and skills. Connecting parents of newly diagnosed children with other more experienced parents who can serve as mentors and information experts is a cherished resource valued by the less experienced parents. Experienced parents of children with SB are viewed uniquely as having the lived experience that adds to their credibility as resource experts. Referrals to community-based parent resource centers provide parents and their families with an array of services that include service coordination, the provision of agency referrals, access to their resource clearinghouse, and advocacy training and services. Studies examining parental needs for supports and services during this stage of their child's development are needed for the development and implementation of evidence-based approaches responsive to these needs.

No studies examining self-management/health have been conducted with parents of preschool-aged children with SB. Knowledge of the child's cognitive, gross motor, fine motor, and visual-perceptual skills serves as the framework for determining the child's level of developmental functioning. Considerable research has been conducted with diverse groups of children to assess their developmental status, as is found in the early intervention literature and follow-up studies of children enrolled in preschool programs such as First Steps and Head Start. However, these studies do not include samples of children with SB. The few studies conducted to assess parental reactions to having a child with SB revealed altered and negative parental perceptions of their child with SB. These perceptions can have detrimental effects on the child's psychosocial and emotional development.[17–19]

A meta-analysis of studies was conducted on parents' adjustment to having a child with SB.[19] The analysis revealed the child's SB had a moderate to large effect on parents' psychological adjustment. The researchers surmised that parents had lower performance expectations for their children with SB compared with typically developing children, thereby expecting the child to perform at a lower level of proficiency compared with typical children of their age. Findings from another study revealed a relationship between parental perception of the child's ability and their reluctance to establish behavioral expectations for their children that fostered self-reliance and self-management.[20]

These findings show the importance of providing parents with anticipatory guidance in fostering the acquisition of self-management skills during this period of development. The initial steps in learning self-management skills are the prerequisite tasks that the child needs to learn to become as independent as possible with their own SB self-management. Clinical programs are based on this assumption of the importance of learning self-management skills. No evaluations of differing approaches to teaching parents management of health have been conducted. The Life Course Model Web site is a tool that can be used both by professionals for self-management instructions for parents and by parents themselves. Evaluation of the strengths and weaknesses of the Web site may add to the literature for younger children.

One study addressed adherence of school-aged children (8–9 years old) with SB.[21] Parents and the child's teacher and physician assessed the child's treatment adherence, referring to their ability to engage in self-management pertaining to the 5 central tasks of SB management: catheterization, bowel care, skin care, medication, and ambulation. Findings revealed that parents reported higher levels of nonadherence, compared with physician and teacher ratings. Children were rated as highest on adherence related to ambulation and lowest on bowel care by parents, physicians, and teachers. The correlations between the rater groups were low and nonsignificant. The lack of agreement was attributed to the variability of the child's behavior across settings as well as the situational differences in the raters' opportunities to observe the children. Researchers found that parents offered several attributions for their children's treatment adherence difficulties. Some parents believed their children were capable but lazy or not motivated to perform self-management tasks; others believed that their children's physical limitations impeded their abilities to adhere to the self-management tasks.

Little is known about HCP expectations for achievement of self-management. Using a list of 25 self-management behaviors of different levels of complexity, Greenley[22] generally found HCPs expected competence in self-management skills for those with moderately severe SB (lumbar lesion, normal intelligence, needing a bowel and bladder program) to be achieved at exit from elementary school or middle school. Children with more severe SB (borderline intelligence, thoracic lesion, using diapers for bowel/bladder program) were expected to achieve skills in high school. No differences were found by HCP type but HCPs seeing more children with SB annually expected tasks to be achieved at an earlier age.

These findings show the importance of assessing parents' and HCPs' perceptions of children's self-management behaviors. Unlike in the earlier years, parents begin to ascribe motivational reasons for the child's self-management behaviors. Parents can be encouraged to use positive reinforcement and refrain from using negative remarks as their children engage in self-management to foster treatment goals. Parents can be encouraged to integrate the child into the daily SB management tasks by using the strategies listed on the Life Course Model Web site.

Adolescents and young adults

Although self-management has been explored in its relationship to level of independence, self-concept, and effect on parents, few studies have been conducted examining self-management in adolescents and young adults with SB. A limited number of studies have examined the relationship of continence and mobility to selected constructs such as self-concept, quality of life, and protective factors. Continence and mobility are indicators of optimal functioning, which are dependent on the individual's ability to competently self-manage their condition.

A study of 60 adolescents with SB aged 12 to 21 years found that their level of lesion was significantly related to their functional status, their level of self-management, and social competence. Although this group of adolescents were found to be fairly independent in functional status, they were less so in SB self-management,[23] especially in advanced skills needed for independent living (eg, ordering supplies, making appointments, performing household chores, managing money, transportation management). In addition, in this same group of adolescents, higher levels of functional status and self-management were significantly associated with adolescents who had household responsibilities compared with those who did not. Neuropsychological status also was a major predictor of functional status[24] and self-management outcomes. Parental expectations for condition-related skills generally were at 17.3 years of age, 2 to 3 years less than independent living skills.[25] These investigators concluded that these independent living skills, especially money management, may be critical precursors to success in employment. Lack of congruency between parent expectations and HCP expectations for select self-management skills suggests a need for more study and intervention.

There are inconsistent findings when examining the relationships of continence and mobility to self-concept and mental health.[26] A study of 24 girls and 26 boys aged 6 to 19 years revealed young people who were continent had significantly higher levels of self-concept, and incontinent girls scored significantly lower in self-concept measures.[27] The findings of this study suggest that incontinence is a socially more sensitive issue for girls in contrast to boys.[27] Other studies found that incontinence was not related to the child's self-concept.[23]

In addition, a synthesis of quality-of-life studies in SB revealed similar inconsistencies.[26] Some investigators found no relationship between continence and health-related quality of life (HRQOL).[28–31] Other investigators, using parent reports and younger children, did find bladder program success related to SB-specific HRQOL.[32] Further, those using an investigator-created HRQOL measure that had continence-specific items found HRQOL increased following bladder surgery.

Researchers studying the emotional effect of CIC on the family (child aged 1–20 years; n = 40) found that raising a child with SB led to strain on the parent-child relationship. This strain adversely affected the emotional component of the parent-child relationship and CIC management.[33] Other studies found that the child's and young person's self-esteem is not adversely affected by CIC issues and may increase the child's level of self-esteem.[34] The effect of continence on mental health and HRQOL needs further study.

Mobility is an important component of self-management and presents a major challenge for many young people with SB. Achievement of optimal mobility enhances multiple outcomes. Low intelligence, hypotonia above the level of the lesion, using a wheelchair for mobility, and poor executive function were noted as significant risk factors for poor self-management skills.[35] However, the role of mobility on self-concept, mental health, and quality of life remains complex. When only the characteristics of SB were evaluated, mobility was found to be the most important determinant for HRQOL for individuals with SB.[35] However, when protective factors such as attitudes, hope, coping, and self-efficacy were included, these psychosocial protective factors had more effect on mental health and quality of life than mobility itself.[28,36]

The other central self-management tasks of SB have not been investigated. No studies were located that examined the factors that enhance or impede shunt management, bowel management, managing skin integrity, weight management, and physical activities.

More study is needed to better understand the self-management needs of children and young people with SB. Researchers have only begun to explore the factors that facilitate or hinder children's/young people's acquisition of self-management skills. Little is known about the most effective strategies to foster the acquisition of the SB self-management skills needed to promote optimal healthy outcomes and prevent and/or minimize the risk of complications and secondary conditions during the period of adolescence. Also needed are studies that delineate the effect of dealing with the hormonal changes of puberty and the developmental tension that exists between independence and continued dependency. The clinical recommendations related to self-management are based on the experience and expertise of clinicians, parents, and individuals with SB. Evidence is needed to inform relevant constituencies of clinical interventions to improve the care for successful acquisition of these skills.

The evidence base related to SB self-management is incomplete, partly because the methodologies used are not comparable. Studies were also limited by use of small convenient sample sizes with unknown biases. Another limitation has been the use of tools with insufficient psychometric properties. In addition, findings about self-management that were associated with specific tasks, such as CIC, were not generalizable to other tasks of SB self-management. More research is needed to better understand the factors that support or inhibit SB self-management. This research should include the use of psychometrically sound instruments with sufficient sample sizes.

Personal/Social Relationships

Gaps in research, programs and services were identified across stages of individual and family development as it pertained to personal/social relationships. The skills needed for effective transition later in life are based on skills developed in early childhood, and the lack of these developmentally appropriate skills puts children with SB at risk. Parents are central to these interventions.

As the Life Course Model Web site was in development, several gaps emerged related to the personal/social domain. First, evidence for interventions that provided parents with effective strategies for developing autonomy and social skills in children with SB was lacking. A second gap pertained to interventions aimed at enhancing resilience in families so that they can provide enhanced support to both their child with SB and other children in the family. These interventions would encompass developing realistic expectations for the child with SB and strategies to facilitate their child's full participation in society.[37–39] Holmbeck and Devine[38] recommended investigating a resilience-disruption theoretic perspective. The third gap involved studies of interventions that increased family understanding of the effect of structural and functional neurologic changes that occur with SB. Specifically, early and ongoing interventions that facilitate identification and remediation of neurologically based executive functioning challenges and the effect of these challenges on peer and family relationships need to be evaluated. The fourth gap was related to parent support programs that focused on building skills of authoritative parenting (ie, providing a mix of structure, affection, and increasing choice to adolescents).

Preschool and school age

Children as young as 3 years of age with SB may lack age-appropriate initiation skills. Clinical programs are needed to support parents in developing a more active approach to facilitate the development of autonomy skills that are like those in typically developing preschool children. Evaluation of programs aimed at increasing choice, increasing age-appropriate responsibility for household chores, and self-care is needed. In addition, although good functional assessment measures exist, practical measures of progressive autonomy need to be developed. The relationship of the level of autonomy skills to socialization skills and peer relationships also needs to be investigated. Evaluating interventions that facilitate development of early socialization skills is also important.

Young people determine their own values and sense of self from those experienced within their family, by peers, or perceived from society's messages as often seen through various media. Along with self-identity, young people are also determining their fit or feelings of belonging to a peer group. Understanding the factors associated with development of self-concept and resilience-based interventions is a priority recommendation.

Adolescence and young adults

The social relationships of young adolescents were studied by Levitt and colleagues,[40] using person-oriented analysis to differentiate patterns of support for children in fourth and sixth grade. Significant shifts in the child's social milieu occurred with the transition from an elementary to a middle-school environment. Self-demands and demands imposed by others for autonomous functioning increased at this time, along with a push/pull toward involvement and identification with a peer group. These researchers reported that children with multiple sources of support were better adjusted than those whose support came primarily from close family members. They reasoned that the availability of alternative sources compensated when close family was not available to meet needs or during times of family conflict. Programs that help young people develop multiple sources of support could provide important sources of protection for young people with SB.

In addition to the normal trials of growing up in an evolving world with parental and peer pressures, children with disabilities must also deal with their disability and the social biases or ignorance that accompanies it. These children are differently able and in some cases markedly so. Late adolescence and emerging adulthood is a time of exploration and finding one's competencies for occupation, relationships, and both independent and interdependent living. It is normally a time for some risk taking. For young people with disabilities, accomplishing the tasks of adolescence and young adulthood is more challenging than for those without disability. Their margin for error may be smaller, the effect of failure perhaps more consequential, and their opportunities for exploration more limited. Few clinical or intervention programs have been conducted to help understand factors that enhance resilience and social skills during this vulnerable time.

For young people with SB, the Life Course Model project emphasized the need for interventions to facilitate social interaction, especially the ability to begin to build reciprocal relationships. Activities that teach the child and parent how to read subtle social cues and provide extensive rehearsal for social interactions are also needed. In addition, interventions/programs to provide children and adolescents with skills necessary for subtle communication and reciprocal relationships with peers are needed.

Also, interventions are needed to teach compensatory strategies for executive functioning challenges because they have an effect on peer and family relationships. Evaluation of programs that (1) facilitate joint problem solving, (2) provide access to new resources, and (3) promote full participation in society is needed. Of special interest are technology-based opportunities to connect with others, as discussed later in the section on employment.

Important programs for school-aged children, adolescents, and young adults exist in limited numbers. Examples are (1) wheelchair sports programs, (2) organizations that promote inclusive recreation and activities, and (3) camps and mentorship programs. Evidence is needed on the effect of these recreational, mentorship, and sports programs in developing social skills, effective self-care skills, and organizational skills.

Studies report that adolescents with SB are at risk for depression,[38,41] with the incidence of anxiety and depression in young adulthood even higher.[42] The limited data indicate that the transition period to adulthood is particular challenging. However, little is known about the risk and protective factors that play an important role in depression or the application of effective interventions to prevent or treat depression in young people with SB. Data from adolescents and young adults suggest that beliefs (attitude, hope, positive coping) are related to the adolescent's report of mental health and that the family influences the development of these resilience beliefs.[23,28,41] Programs that enhance resilience skills need to be developed and tested. These interventions may be especially important for young people whose family has limited financial or family resources.

Another programmatic and knowledge gap identified in the Life Course Model project was relationships with siblings. We need to better understand the needs of both the young people with SB and their siblings and provide services to both. Research has shown both the positive effect and the challenges for siblings of young people with SB.[43,44] However, little is known about the effect of sibling programs (eg, Sibshops) on the sibling and family.

The personal and social relationship gaps identified in the development of this Life Course Model project are consistent with a recent review of the psychosocial research in SB by Holmbeck and Devine.[38] These investigators suggest that future research should address 3 overall priorities: (1) evaluate longitudinal models of psychosocial outcomes and particularly investigate mediators of outcomes; (2) identify individual, family, and parenting factors that explain success in emerging adulthood for young people with SB; and (3) identify resilience factors associated with successful outcomes in young people with SB and their families.

Employment/Income Support

Characteristics of SB and academic achievement are both precursors to employment success. Despite some descriptive studies, the relationship of spinal lesion level, brain, and adaptive behavioral differences to outcome is not well understood.[23,29,45,46] The efficacy of interventions designed to promote independence and productivity has yet to be clearly shown.

Characteristics of SB

The lives of individuals with SB are complex and the challenges multifactorial. An understanding of the natural history of individuals with SB across the life course is only now emerging. Technological and health care developments in recent years have offered potential for longer, fuller, healthier lives. This potential is yet to be fully realized at each developmental stage across the life course. Assessment of the individual and environmental factors and the implementation of interventions at critical periods, particularly at key transition points such as preschool to school, junior high to high school, graduation, transition from pediatric to adult health care, and moving from home to less supervised living arrangements, offer opportunities for reconsideration and implementation of new strategies.[23,47,48]

Performance patterns across the lesion-level subgroups revealed that the lesion level had a greater effect on motor than cognitive function, although both domains were affected. The high rates of learning and attention disabilities may lead to more adverse outcomes in terms of social communication and community living.[45] Future studies on effective strategies to advance functional performance within and across the domains of health, education, employment, and community participation should incorporate a longitudinal view to determine if acquisition of discrete skills, such as balancing a checkbook, monitoring the condition of skin, transferring independently, or driving, translates into an improved life trajectory as measured by academic achievement, independence, employment, health, and personal/social relationships.

Although mobility is a predictor of employment, little has been published regarding its effect on independence and employment. Assistive technology use among adolescents and young adults with SB may influence achievement of independence, academic achievement, and employment, yet little research has been carried out to determine the frequency of assistive technology use and its effectiveness on outcomes for individuals with SB. The more traditional technology applications for mobility, such as crutches, walkers, and wheelchairs, have been found to increase the risk of upper-extremity damage. This musculoskeletal stress and strain could have an effect on longer-term self-care and mobility. So there is a gap in our understanding of the long-term implications of the various modalities of mobility. In a focus group sponsored by the Spina Bifida Association in 2010, working adults with SB regretted pushing themselves so hard physically because they experienced later pain and fatigue. Assistive technologies such as smart phones, personal data assistants, and miniaturized recorders are experiencing a higher level of social acceptance. Maintenance, cost, and other factors, such as the need for setup and training, may be barriers to use of assistive technologies for individuals with SB. Johnson and colleagues[49] stated that using assistive technology can result in significantly enhanced independence, employment, and life satisfaction. Study is needed to determine which assistive technologies can contribute across the lifespan, across a broader range of performance domains, and to determine what protections are needed to miti-gate negative secondary effects from their use.[49]

Academic achievement

Current theory, as articulated by Jaffari-Bimmel and colleagues[50] in 2006, concurs with Erikson's step-wise or building-block approach. "Development is the interplay between a changing environment and a changing individual, but early experiences and adaptations do not fade away. Instead, they indirectly shape future adaptation through their influences on intermediary developmental steps."[(p1150)] Bronstein and colleagues'[51] study provided evidence that parental behavior may affect children's motivation during the transition to middle school by fostering academic performance and sense of scholastic competence. These investigators found academic success led to children having more positive perceptions of their scholastic competence, leading to the development of an intrinsic motivational orientation. Poorer academic performance led to self-perception that was more negative and to the development of a more extrinsic motivational orientation. Autonomy-supporting parental behaviors such as allowing children to express their ideas and opinions and to participate in family decisions may have helped develop the children's capacity for independent thinking and problem solving[51] (see also the section on personal/social relationships). This encouragement for independent thinking, problem solving, and self-efficacy–promoted achievement may stimulate inquiry to better understand factors that influ-ence the child's level of functioning.

Employment

Previous research on work participation generally showed overall rates of employment between 19% and 38%. Predictors of having paid work (at least 1 hour a week) were level of education, level of lesion, hydrocephalus, IQ, self-care independence, and ambulation.

In the study by van Mechelen and colleagues,[52] bowel and bladder continence made it 2.5 times more likely for the individual with SB to be employed. A higher level of education was an important and positive indicator of employment. Another study found lower levels of post-secondary education, with 41%–49% of individuals with SB attending college vs 66% of typically developing young people[38] which may have a major effect on underemployment.

Van Mechelen and colleagues[52] also found that the most effective time to help young people find a job was immediately after they finished their education, noting that motivation to work would gradually decrease once they accepted welfare bene-fits. Young adults with SB who had experienced problems in finding suitable employ-ment reported difficulties, with reluctant attitudes among employers (57%), work offered that was physically (30%) or mentally (27%) too demanding, transportation (32%), accessibility of buildings (23%), and toilet space (23%). To date most studies have focused on either demographic or condition severity factors as predictors of employment success. Understanding individual, family, environmental, and financial factors associated with successful completion of higher education should also be studied. These factors might include lack of autonomy-related socialization,[53,54] accessibility and transportation difficulties, insurance complexities, stigma, and lack of job training.[38,55,56]

Reiss and colleagues'[57] research identified 3 stages of transition: envisioning the future, age of responsibility, and age of transition. Children with disabilities need encouragement to envision their future. Assessment and intervention approaches to facilitate independence and readiness for employment should be appropriate for the individual's age and stage of development.

Preschool and school-aged children

Early intervention programs for infants and toddlers exist throughout the United States and almost universally children with SB qualify for these services. Evidence is lacking about the interventions in these programs that improve mobility, overall development, and efficient transition to school-based programs.

Difficulties in language, learning, memory, and attention emerge during this time. There is limited evidence regarding when to perform neuropsychological assessment of these skills. Individuals with SB and their parents or caregivers have expressed a lack of awareness with not only the terminology but also the concepts of executive function and nonlearning disabilities. A few programs for preschool children have developed mechanisms to systematically evaluate executive, attention, and learning functions.[58] These programs, aimed at children with various disabilities[59] including SB, focus on developing compensatory skills at an early age. Because these programs offer the opportunity for early intervention, their evaluation should be a high priority.

Programs that institute early testing for core neuropsychological processing skills are needed in the early elementary years. Studies evaluating age-appropriate interventions and accommodation strategies (especially for mathematics) are needed to optimize early school success. Autonomy skills may be limited by these core neuropsychological skills (see section on personal/social relationships). Evidence of the most effective, age-appropriate, reality-based interventions to increase function in areas such as managing money, planning and organizing, and solving real life problems should be evaluated. Evaluation of technology to organize, support, and prompt behavior in both school and self-care activities is needed.

Adolescents

Evidence is lacking of the optimal structure and components of an effective transition plan that addresses the critical areas for students who have an Individualized Education Plan. In 1999 to 2000, the standard diploma graduation rate for students with disabilities aged 14 years and older was 56.2%. During the same period, the dropout rate declined from 34.1% to 29.4%.[60] Graduation from high school and/or postsecondary education programs leading to employment are key factors in attaining the highest level of autonomy.

Attaining meaningful employment that reflects the preferences and interests of the individual with disabilities is too important to be left to chance. Careful planning, dedication of resources, and educational programming are essential to achieving this goal. Because of the marked disadvantages for young people with disabilities when competing for employment, opportunities for career exploration and skill building should occur before the young person is placed in a specific program. Assessment of aptitudes, special needs, learning style, personal and social skills, values, and attitudes toward work as well as work tolerance can assist the student to learn about himself or herself and inform their career choices.[61] The effectiveness of work-related programs offered in high schools to build self-management, social skills, and work behaviors needs to be evaluated. Access to and the effectiveness of vocational rehabilitation/career counseling interventions needs to be assessed in terms of assisting students with SB to obtain postsecondary employment.

Young adults

Material consequences, pay for performance, and other social rewards and privileges are common motivators. Individuals regulate their own behavior by self-evaluative and other self-produced consequences.[62] If an individual is unable to earn material rewards or experience positive recognition and acknowledgment of accomplishment, their sense of self may suffer. The long-term implications of diminished self-confidence and self-esteem need more study.

Programs that provide coordination for posthigh-school skills, supportive employment, or transition to postsecondary education need to be developed and evaluated. Especially important is delineating the components of these programs that are the most effective in predicting employment, quality of life, and community participation outcomes.

Across domains and life course

Executive function challenges and nonverbal learning differences are 2 conditions that can greatly affect how an individual with SB does in life. A person's executive function system is responsible for self-awareness and the ability to plan and carry out tasks in daily life. It modulates both emotions and behavior. Learning disorders are caused by a difference in the brain that affects how information is received, processed, or communicated. The expressive verbal skills and social nature of people with SB may conceal nonverbal challenges.

A learning disability is not a problem with intelligence. Individuals with learning disabilities have difficulty processing sensory information because they see, hear, and understand things differently. Advancements in the science of how the brain adapts, through a process called neuroplasticity, suggests a natural, lifelong ability to form new connections and generate new brain cells in response to experience and learning. Opportunities to affect learning and executive function by retraining the brain may hold promise for reorganizing neuronal connections and facilitate skill-building capabilities for individuals with SB. Application of the science of neuroplasticity to individuals with SB, particularly those with hydrocephalus, is an exciting area for future research. Training (repetitive practice for skill building) offers a different way of facilitating learning, compared with teaching (telling once or twice), a method commonly used in academic, employment, and health care settings.

SUMMARY AND PRIORITY RECOMMENDATIONS

The Life Course Model project has identified that little progress has been made on the research agenda priorities generated after the 2003 consensus conference on SB (see **Table 1**). Gaps persist in the knowledge, programs, and services across individual and family developmental stages that need to be addressed to facilitate transition in self-management/health, personal and social relationships, and employment/income support. Research is needed that is theory-driven (model testing), longitudinal, addresses critical developmental periods or transition points, is inclusive of ethnic and socioeconomic diversity, is multisite and with sufficient sample size to address multiple variables, and identifies the trajectory of SB across the life course.

Furthermore, studies are needed that move from identifying differences between those chronic health conditions, like SB, and typically developing peers to addressing why the differences occur. Studies that identify personal, family, and environmental factors associated with successful achievement of self-management/health, personal and social relationships, and employment and interventions based on these factors are immediate priorities for optimizing the successful transition to adulthood. The effect of successful employment experiences on social and quality-of-life outcomes needs to be investigated.

The 3 domains defined in the Life Course Model have natural overlaps that need more study. For instance, how do cognitive skills affect self-management and personal/social relationships? We also need to determine if there are critical time points at which intervention might make a difference in the trajectory and outcomes. Valid and reliable measurement of the milestones depicted in the Life Course Model is also a challenge. The commonly used and available instruments may not be appropriate for measurement of important constructs. With so many more adults living with SB, they should be used to identify important proximal and distal outcomes, develop research questions, and validate measures. A collaborative partnership with all stakeholders offers the most promise of enhancing the science and improving the lives of all living with SB.

REFERENCES

1. Liptak G, editor. Evidence-based practice in spina bifida: developing a research agenda. Washington, DC: Spina Bifida Association; 2003.
2. Liptak G, editor. First World Congress on Spina Bifida Research and Care Proceedings. Washington, DC: Spina Bifida Association; 2009.
3. Fletcher JM, Brei TJ. Introduction: spina bifida–a multidisciplinary perspective. Dev Disabil Res Rev 2010;16(1):1–5.
4. Merkens M, editor. Guidelines for spina bifida health care services throughout the lifespan. Washington, DC: Spina Bifida Association; 2006.
5. World Heath Organization. International classification of functioning, disability, and health. Geneva (Switzerland): World Health Organization; 2001.
6. Greenley RN. A family intervention to enhance involvement in condition management of youth with spina bifida: a pilot study. Scientific abstracts: the future is now. Orlando (FL): First World Congress on Spina Bifida Research and Care; 2009.
7. Holmbeck GN, Greenley RN, Coakley RM, et al. Family functioning in children and adolescents with spina bifida: an evidence-based review of research and interventions. J Dev Behav Pediatr 2006;27(3):249–77.
8. Dennis M, Landry SH, Barnes M, et al. A model of neurocognitive function in spina bifida over the life span. J Int Neuropsychol Soc 2006;12(2):285–96.
9. Sellet S. Creating tele learning communities and social networks or teens and young adults with spina bifida. Scientific Abstracts: The Future is Now. First World Congress on Spina Bifida Research and Care. Orlando (FL): Spina Bifida Association; 2009.
10. Rauen K. Mentoring projects for teens with spina bifida result in improved socialization skills, independence and community participation. Scientific Abstracts. The Future is Now. First World Congress on Spina Bifida Research and Care. Orlando (FL): Spina Bifida Association; 2009.
11. Aldana PR, Ragheb J, Sevald J, et al. Cerebrospinal fluid shunt complications after urological procedures in children with myelodysplasia. Neurosurgery 2002;50(2):313–8.
12. Greenley RN, Coakley RM, Holmbeck GN, et al. Condition-related knowledge among children with spina bifida: longitudinal changes and predictors. J Pediatr Psychol 2006;31(8):828–39.
13. Hetherington R, Dennis M, Barnes M, et al. Functional outcome in young adults with spina bifida and hydrocephalus. Childs Nerv Syst 2006;22(2):117–24.
14. McDonnell GV, McCann JP. Why do adults with spina bifida and hydrocephalus die? A clinic-based study. Eur J Pediatr Surg 2000;1:31–2.
15. Oakeshott P, Hunt GM. Long-term outcome in open spina bifida. Br J Gen Pract 2003;53(493):632–6.
16. Hunt G, Oakeshott P, Kerry S. Link between the CSF shunt and achievement in adults with spina bifida. J Neurol Neurosurg Psychiatry 1999;67(5):591–5.

17. Blaymore Bier JA, Liebling JA, Morales Y, et al. Parents' and pediatricians' views of individuals with meningomyelocele. Clin Pediatr (Phila) 1996;35(3):113–7.
18. Vachha B, Adams RC. Memory and selective learning in children with spina bifida-myelomeningocele and shunted hydrocephalus: a preliminary study. Cerebrospinal Fluid Res 2005;2:10.
19. Vermaes IP, Janssens JM, Bosman AM, et al. Parents' psychological adjustment in families of children with spina bifida: a meta-analysis. BMC Pediatr 2005;5:32.
20. Vachha B, Adams R. Influence of family environment on language outcomes in children with myelomeningocele. Child Care Health Dev 2005;31(5):589–96.
21. Holmbeck GN, Belvedere MC, Christensen M, et al. Assessment of adherence with multiple informants in pre-adolescents with spina bifida: initial development of a multidimensional, multitask parent-report questionnaire. J Pers Assess 1998; 70(3):427–40.
22. Greenley RN. Health professional expectations for self-care skill development in youth with spina bifida. Pediatr Nurs 2010;36(2):98–102.
23. Sawin KJ, Buran CF, Brei TJ, et al. Correlates of functional status, self-management, and developmental competence outcomes in adolescents with spina bifida. SCI Nurs 2003;20(2):72–85.
24. Heffelfinger AK, Koop JI, Fastenau PS, et al. The relationship of neuropsychological functioning to adaptation outcome in adolescents with spina bifida. J Int Neuropsychol Soc 2008;14(5):793–804.
25. Sawin KJ, Brei TJ. Enhancing independence. Dublin (Ireland): World Congress, Next Steps, International Federation of Spina Bifida and Hydrocephalus; 2010.
26. Sawin KJ, Bellin MH. Quality of life in individuals with spina bifida: a research update. Dev Disabil Res Rev 2010;16:47–59.
27. Moore C, Kogan BA, Parekh A. Impact of urinary incontinence on self-concept in children with spina bifida. J Urol 2004;171(4):1659–62.
28. Sawin KJ, Brei TJ, Buran CF, et al. Factors associated with quality of life in adolescents with spina bifida. J Holist Nurs 2002;20(3):279–304.
29. Leger RR. Severity of illness, functional status, and HRQOL in youth with spina bifida. including commentary by Zimmerman B. Rehabil Nurs 2005;30(5): 180–8.
30. Parekh AD, Trusler LA, Pietsch JB, et al. Prospective, longitudinal evaluation of health related quality of life in the pediatric spina bifida population undergoing reconstructive urological surgery. J Urol 2006;176(4 Pt 2):1878–82.
31. Lemelle JL, Guillemin F, Aubert D, et al. Quality of life and continence in patients with spina bifida. Qual Life Res 2006;15(9):1481–92.
32. Brand J, Sawin KJ, Koo H, et al. Urologic outcomes and quality of life in children with a neurogenic bladder: a pilot study. Scientific Abstracts: The Future is Now. First World Congress on Spina Bifida Research and Care. Orlando (FL): Spina Bifida Association; 2009.
33. Borzyskowski M, Cox A, Edwards M, et al. Neuropathic bladder and intermittent catheterization: social and psychological impact on families. Dev Med Child Neurol 2004;46(3):160–7.
34. Edwards M, Borzyskowski M, Cox A, et al. Neuropathic bladder and intermittent catheterization: social and psychological impact on children and adolescents. Dev Med Child Neurol 2004;46(3):168–77.
35. Schoenmakers MA, Uiterwaal CS, Gulmans VA, et al. Determinants of functional independence and quality of life in children with spina bifida. Clin Rehabil 2005; 19(6):677–85.

36. Kirpalani HM, Parkin PC, Willan AR, et al. Quality of life in spina bifida: importance of parental hope. Arch Dis Child 2000;83(4):293–7.
37. Singh DK. Families of children with spina bifida: a review. J Dev Phys Disabil 2003;15:37–55.
38. Holmbeck GN, Devine KA. Psychosocial and family functioning in spina bifida. Dev Disabil Res Rev 2010;16:40–6.
39. Kazak AE, Simms S, Barakat L, et al. Surviving Cancer Competently Intervention Program (SCCIP): a cognitive-behavioral and family therapy intervention for adolescent survivors of childhood cancer and their families. Fam Process 1999;38(2):175–91.
40. Levitt M, Levitt J, Bustos G, et al. Patterns of social support in the middle childhood to early adolescent transition: implications for adjustment. Soc Dev 2005; 14(3):398–420.
41. Brei TJ, Sawin KJ, Webb T, et al. Testing a model predicting health related quality of life in a multi-site study of adolescents & young adults with spina bifida. Scientific abstracts: the future is now. First World Congress on Spina Bifida Research and Care. Orlando (FL): Spina Bifida Association; 2009.
42. Bellin MH, Zabel TA, Dicianno B, et al. Correlates of depressive and anxiety symptoms in young adults with spina bifida. J Pediatr Psychol 2010;35(7): 778–89.
43. Bellin MH, Bentley KJ, Sawin KJ. Factors associated with the psychological and behavioral adjustment of siblings of youths with spina bifida. Fam Syst Health 2009;27(1):1–15.
44. Bellin MH, Kovacs PJ, Sawin KJ. Risk and protective influences in the lives of siblings of youths with spina bifida. Health Soc Work 2008;33(3):199–209.
45. Fletcher JM, Copeland K, Frederick JA, et al. Spinal lesion level in spina bifida: a source of neural and cognitive heterogeneity. J Neurosurg 2005;102(Suppl 3):268–79.
46. Verhoef M, Barf HA, Post MW, et al. Secondary impairments in young adults with spina bifida. Dev Med Child Neurol 2004;46(6):420–7.
47. Zabel TA, Ries J, Mahone EM, et al. The Kennedy Independence Scales-Spina Bifida version: a parent report rating scale of adaptive functioning in adolescents with spina bifida. Eur J Pediatr Surg 2003;13(Suppl 1):S37–9.
48. Betz CL, Redcay G, Tan S. Self-reported health care needs of transition-age youth: a pilot study. Issues Compr Pediatr Nurs 2003;26(3):159–91.
49. Johnson KL, Dudgeon B, Kuehn C, et al. Assistive technology use among adolescents and young adults with spina bifida. Am J Public Health 2007; 97(2):330–6.
50. Jaffari-Bimmel N, Juffer F, van Ijzendoom M, et al. Social development from infancy to adolescence: longitudinal and concurrent factors in an adoption sample. Dev Psychol 2006;46(6):1143–53.
51. Bronstein P, Ginsburg G, Herrera I. Parental predictors of motivational orientation in early adolescence: a longitudinal study. J Youth Adolesc 2005;34(6):559–75.
52. van Mechelen MC, Verhoef M, van Asbeck FW, et al. Work participation among young adults with spina bifida in the Netherlands. Dev Med Child Neurol 2008; 50(10):772–7.
53. Dicianno BE, Gaines A, Collins DM, et al. Mobility, assistive technology use, and social integration among adults with spina bifida. Am J Phys Med Rehabil 2009; 88(7):533–41.
54. Dicianno BE, Bellin MH, Zabel AT. Spina bifida and mobility in the transition years. Am J Phys Med Rehabil 2009;88(12):1002–6.

55. Buran CF, McDaniel AM, Brei TJ. Needs assessment in a spina bifida program: a comparison of the perceptions by adolescents with spina bifida and their parents. Clin Nurse Spec 2002;16(5):256–62.
56. Barf HA, Post MW, Verhoef M, et al. Restrictions in social participation of young adults with spina bifida. Disabil Rehabil 2009;31(11):921–7.
57. Reiss J, Gibson R, Walker L. Health care transition: youth, family, and provider perspectives. Pediatrics 2005;115:112–20.
58. Heffelfinger A, Koop J. A description of the neuropsychological assessment and diagnostic impressions in the P.I.N.T. clinic after the first five years. Clin Neuropsychol 2009;23:51–76.
59. Heffelfinger A, Craft S, White D, et al. Visual attention in preschool children prenatally exposed to cocaine: implications for behavioral regulation. J Int Neuropsychol Soc 2002;8:12–21.
60. Office of Special Education Programs. 24th Annual Report to Congress on the Implementation of IDEA. Washington, DC: US Government Printing Office; 2001.
61. National Information Center for Children and Youth with Disabilities. Transition summary: vocational assessment: a guide for parents and professionals. Washington, DC: National Information Center for Children and Youth with Disabilities; 1990.
62. Bandura A. Social learning theory. Englewood Cliffs (NJ): Prentice-Hall; 1977.

Index

Note: Page numbers of article titles are in **boldface** type.

Pediatr Clin N Am 57 (2010) 1059–1068
doi:10.1016/S0031-3955(10)00125-2
0031-3955/10/$ – see front matter

Moving?

Make sure your subscription moves with you!

To notify us of your new address, find your **Clinics Account Number** (located on your mailing label above your name), and contact customer service at:

Email: journalscustomerservice-usa@elsevier.com

800-654-2452 (subscribers in the U.S. & Canada)
314-447-8871 (subscribers outside of the U.S. & Canada)

Fax number: 314-447-8029

Elsevier Health Sciences Division
Subscription Customer Service
3251 Riverport Lane
Maryland Heights, MO 63043